WALKING CHICAGO

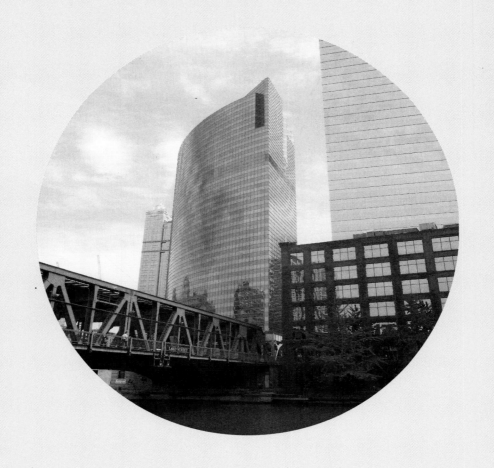

WALKING CHICAGO

31 tours of the Windy City's
classic bars, scandalous sites, historic
architecture, dynamic neighborhoods,
and famous lakeshore

Ryan Ver Berkmoes

 WILDERNESS PRESS · BERKELEY, CA

917.7311
VER

Walking Chicago: 31 tours of the Windy City's classic bars, scandalous sites, historic architecture, dynamic neighborhoods, and famous lakeshore

1st EDITION September 2008

Cover photos copyright © 2008 by Ryan Ver Berkmoes
Interior photos: Ryan Ver Berkmoes, except p. 63, courtesy Mary Ann Bryan, www.beverlymorganpark.net
Maps: Bart Wright/Fineline Maps
Book and cover design: Larry B. Van Dyke
Book editor: Marc Lecard
Copyeditor: Jan Caroll
Layout: Beverly Butterfield, Girl of the West Productions

ISBN 978-0-89997-416-3

Manufactured in Canada

Published by: **Wilderness Press**
                  1345 8th Street
                  Berkeley, CA 94710
                  (800) 443-7227; FAX (510) 558-1696
                  info@wildernesspress.com
                  www.wildernesspress.com

Visit our website for a complete listing of our books and for ordering information.

Cover photos: *Front, clockwise from upper right: Cloud Gate* (a.k.a. "The Bean"), Millennium Park; Erie St. Park; gracious Victorian home in Andersonville; the Green Mill, Uptown; looking northeast from Sears Tower; Frank Lloyd Wright–designed home, Oak Park. *Back, clockwise from upper right: Agora,* by Magdalena Abakanowicz; farmers market in front of the Museum of Contemporary Art; Robie House.

Frontispiece: The iconic 333 Wacker Building, on the Riverwalk

SAFETY NOTICE: Although Wilderness Press and the author have made every attempt to ensure that the information in this book is accurate at press time, they are not responsible for any loss, damage, injury, or inconvenience that may occur to anyone while using this book. You are responsible for your own safety and health while following the walking trips described here. Always check local conditions, know your own limitations, and consult a map.

acknowledgments

Where to start? I am lucky enough to have a group of friends who I've not only gone for a lot of walks with in Chicago, but who were enthusiastic about this book from the start. In no order: John Holden is a walking encyclopedia on the city; Howard Larkin is as good a walking companion as you could hope for; Susan and Chris Amati are wonderful walking companions (note subtle diplomatic difference). Yucking it up from Obama's to Veeck's, Sandy Eitel has barely tapped research skills and could replace me at this, but don't tell her. Kelly McGrath was there the first night and the last; Ed Mazur brings new insight to Victor Mature and vast swaths of the city; Ed Lawler does the same for Beverly; Margaret Fosmoe kept me on track (now and in the past); James Borkman is my new official biographer; and Erin Corrigan made the dreams of the Gold Coast a dream. Others vital to happy walking and authoring: Pat Byrnes, Kate Campion, Janice Chambers, Bill & Alicia Derrah, Lisa Donovan, Dave Fell, Darel Jevens, Rick Kogan, Leo Burns and Mary Ann O'Rourke, Kathleen Pratt, Mark Rust and his iPod-deserving family, Nancy Ryan, author Lawrence P. Santoro, Mark Stewart, Becky Voelker, the incomparable Karla Zimmerman, Christine Zrinsky (who helped with some of the photos) and Roslyn Bullas, who sent the email that launched this project in the first place.

author's note

Chicago is a wonderful city for walking for two reasons: a) it's flat as a board, and b) it's hard to get lost. You truly have to pound the pavement to work up a sweat most of year (excepting certain summer months when doing nothing can leave you drenched). And the street layout, with addresses that always include a north, south, east, or west, functions as an inherent GPS. Plus you can always remember the mantra: "The lake is east. The lake is east."

The walks in this book have been chosen to allow you to explore the city in ways that even grizzled natives will find at times surprising. Concerns about personal safety and the character of neighborhoods are common for locals, whether justified or not. And some neighborhoods in this book have not always enjoyed the most sterling of reputations. But generally, during the day and with a few street smarts (if a corner looks dodgy, avoid it; skip the lonely alleys, etc.), you should be fine and be able to enjoy parts of Chicago often untrod. Bring friends, as there's always reassurance in numbers, and you'll have more fun sharing the experience.

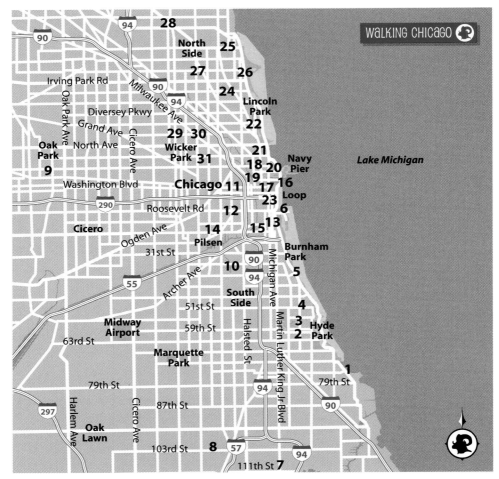

Numbers on this locator map correspond to Walk numbers.

TABLE OF CONTENTS

INTRODUCTION

Can there be a better city for walking than Chicago? Neighborhoods reeking with character (some literally), a history that would be great fiction if it weren't true, stirring architecture, 21 miles of lakefront, and parks worthy of an empire. If it's not flat enough for you, there are several hundred good joints to plop down in and re-energize—and maybe have a touch of refreshment.

Walking in Chicago, you realize what a dynamic place it is. Every block yields a new surprise, discovery, or quirk. Every step leads to a unique view, whether it's the soaring skyline seen from the lakefront or some tiny bit of urban drama glimpsed from the sidewalk. Follow the Chicago River and you encounter one new building after another—for better or worse. Prowl the streets of classic neighborhoods like Bridgeport, Little Italy and Wicker Park to see their very fabric changing right before your eyes.

Walking brings you close to the dreams of Chicagoans here and gone. Grand, cathedral-sized churches built for the ages by congregations that no longer exist are next door to small shops where families are just beginning their climb up the ladder. The city's experience hasn't been focus-grouped or market-tested. Rather, it's there for you to take as you will, letting your own moods, interests and reactions shape your experience.

This book's 31 walks span the city from the far south to the very north, from Oak Park in the west to the lakefront in the east. Difficulty of terrain doesn't play a factor in a city where the highest hills are usually curbs; you can follow right along as Chicago reinvents itself block by block with nothing to hinder your wanderings. New, old, rich, poor, beautiful, ugly, famous and infamous—it's all here. Choose a walk at random or with deliberation; maybe I'll bump into you around the next corner.

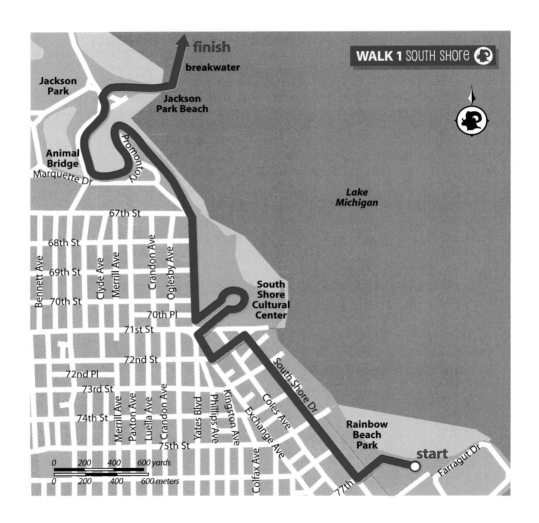

WALK 1 SOUTH SHORE

finish

breakwater

Jackson Park

Jackson Park Beach

Animal Bridge

Marquette Dr

Promontory

67th St

68th St

Bennett Ave

69th St

Clyde Ave

Merrill Ave

70th St

Crandon Ave

Oglesby Ave

70th Pl

71st St

Lake Michigan

South Shore Cultural Center

72nd St

72nd Pl

73rd St

Merrill Ave

Paxton Ave

Luella Ave

Crandon Ave

74th St

Yates Blvd

Phillips Ave

Kingston Ave

Exchange Ave

75th St

Coles Ave

Colfax Ave

South Shore Dr

Rainbow Beach Park

start

Farragut Dr

77th

0   200   400   600 yards
0   200   400   600 meters

1 SOUTH SHOPE: LaKeFRONT GENTILITY

BOUNDARIES: Jackson Park, Lake Michigan, E. 79th St., S. South Shore Dr.
DISTANCE: 4.7 miles (one way)
PUBLIC TRANSIT: Metra Electric to Cheltenham stop; 6 Jackson Park Express bus

Never as toney as other lakeside neighborhoods, South Shore has long been a middle-class refuge featuring excellent lakeshore views (the land bulging east means that you can easily look north to the bright lights of downtown). Many of the buildings date from the 1920s and 1930s when this neighborhood was home to a mix of white Protestants, Catholics and Jews. Like so many other parts of the city, South Shore had a deeply troubled racial transformation in the 1950s and 1960s, including riots at its beaches. Ironically, little has changed since the 1940s except the color of the residents' skin. South Shore makes for a good lakeside walk. Revitalized park facilities take advantage of the stunning locations, and the community's genteel roots are fully on display. In addition you can find surprises like one of Chicago's many Blues Brothers locations and several now tranquil beaches for getting your feet wet. The walk touches on Jackson Park.

● Start at the 67-acre Rainbow Beach Park, which has an entrance at the east end of E. 79th St. This long crescent of sand is one of the city's finest beaches. Today, the water is clean and the air clear by city standards, but before the 1990s, the US Steel South Works sprawled across the now empty land south of the park. Until it closed in 1992, the plant belched pollution of all forms out of its pipes. It also employed more than 20,000 people at its peak. The surrounding area has never recovered from the economic blow of Big Steel's departure.

The entrance to Rainbow Beach is dominated by what looks like a minimum-security prison. In reality, this is a water-filtration plant that supplies drinking water sourced from structures called "cribs" (so-named before the rap generation co-opted the term), located several miles out in the lake. This keeps the industrial pollution and sewage that were once dumped into the lake with abandon from pouring out of the city's faucets. The center of the beach is the small but smart beach house, which opened in 2000. Note the whimsical, cloud-shaped glass awnings. Numerous special activities keep the park filled with kids throughout the year. On summer weekends, the shady expanses of lawn are alive with family groups barbecuing. It's a festival of Moo & Oink, Chicago's legendary chain of supermarkets that cater to the mega-cookout crowds.

- Walk north along the beach and note the patches of dune grass amidst the rolling sand.

- Look for some low-rise structures through the trees to the northwest, away from the shore, and cut across the grass to roughly where E. 77th St. would intersect the park. The buildings here are part of a park district fitness center. Listen for breathless shouts and taunts, and you'll find the three outdoor handball courts, the only ones of their kind in the city. Here, a mixed crowd of hardy souls can be found banging rubber balls with competitive ferocity throughout most of the year.

- Head north along S. South Shore Dr. The park ends at E. 75th St. and streets from here to E. 71st St. all dead-end at the lake. The buildings are a mixture of classic high-rise apartments from the 1920s and the more architecturally modest efforts of the 1960s.

- At 72nd St., turn left to walk two blocks west, past some tidy three-flats to the corner of S. Exchange Ave. Here, the Exchange Cafe offers the best refreshments you'll find on the walk. Try a panini sandwich or a shot of espresso to put some lead in your tank for the rest of the walk.

- Walk north one long block along S. Exchange Ave. Down the middle of the street run the tracks of Metra's South Chicago branch. The double-decker electric trains are unique to the system and reach the Loop in less than 30 minutes.

- At the busy intersection of Exchange, E. 71st St., and S. South Shore Dr., cross to the northeast corner and enter the 65-acre grounds of the South Shore Cultural Center, which includes a grand old dame of a building decked out in maroon that serves as both a community performance and events space and as a clubhouse for an immaculate, par-33, nine-hole golf course. The complex has roots as the South Side Country Club, an exclusionary institution that was started for rich whites in 1905. The present building dates from 1916, when Marshall and Fox, a firm known for their high-end work for Chicago's elite, designed the Mediterranean fantasy you see today. However, all was almost lost in the 1970s when the original club failed, its roster depleted and surviving members unwilling to allow in the South Shore's middle-class African-American residents. The Chicago Park District saved the site from demolition, restored the principal structures and rechristened it as a cultural center.

As you enter the dual, colonnaded, gabled entry, you'll first smell and then see the stables. These are used by the Chicago Police Department for their mounted patrols—a feature of present-day parades as well as past events like the 1968 Democratic Convention riots. Inside the clubhouse, the decor is downscale grandluxe. The north ballroom is a gem of frills and glass, and there are fine views across the lake; the furnishings themselves are strictly for the masses. Outside there's plenty to see, even for non-lawn-fetishists and golfers. If the front façade looks familiar, it may be because the clubhouse exterior was used as the "Palace Hotel," the place Jake and Elwood first performed in the *Blues Brothers*. The beach, sheltered by the clubhouse and fairways, is a long, curving dream with a small native plant display.

● Exit the South Shore Cultural Center and walk north along S. South Shore Dr. This is the most upscale part of the neighborhood, with high-rises on the west side occupied by some of African-American Chicago's bourgeoisie. Especially on weekends, look for golfers stepping out in extravagant duds.

● At E. 67th St., where the golf course fence ends, walk north on the sidewalk that becomes a waterfront path. Getting away from the busy streets, this isthmus gets increasingly

Rainbow Beach

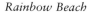

peaceful even if it's not particularly well groomed. The complex of buildings 600 yards north of E. 67th St. is La Rabida Children's Hospital, which is dedicated to helping kids with chronic illnesses or disabilities. The serene lakefront setting is ideal for the institution's mission and was home to Spain's pavilion during the 1893 Columbian Exhibition. The pavilion was modeled after the La Rabida Convent, where Columbus purportedly waited for Ferdinand and Isabella's decision about his trip in search of India. Today's buildings are modern inside and take design cues from the long-demolished faux convent.

Continue past the hospital to the point of the isthmus. From the circular path at the tip, you can look across the channel to Jackson Park Beach, your ultimate goal.

● Walk back south along the west side of the Isthmus. In temperate months you'll see tall-masted yachts belonging to members of the Jackson Park Yacht Club. Founded in 1896, the club's initial dues were $1. But the cost to members was often far more. Although the club was located on a channel dug for the Columbian Exposition, below the waters lurked an ocean of peril. When the fair ended, workers tossed vast amounts of debris into the water. Boaters could easily come to grief, say, by getting speared on the spire of a cast-off funhouse. But yachters had clout then, too, and dredging soon began and continues to this day (sand would otherwise quickly block the entrance).

● Follow the waterside path west around the north side of E. Marquette Dr., and then turn north to cross the beautifully restored Animal Bridge over the entrance to the motorboat docking basin. Take a moment to look at the profusion of animal heads adorning the sides of the bridge; critters include hippos, rhinos, and an angry goat. From the wide sidewalk along the water, you can look across to the yacht club and La Rabida. The shingled complex of wooden buildings that look like something out of a summertime lake fantasy are part of the former Coast Guard Station, which was built in 1906. It's been nicely restored and is used by the park district.

● Cross behind the old Coast Guard Station and continue along the waterfront walk until you come to the wide swath of sand that is Jackson Park Beach, one of the most formal and attractive beaches in Chicago. The classic beach house dates from 1919 and was designed by the old parks commission to incorporate Mediterranean details as well as taking its cues from some of Daniel Burnham's work. A lavish restoration in 1999 included special work on the extensive courtyards, which were gathering spots for bathers back in the days when a trip to the beach could be a surprisingly formal affair. Note that in some quarters, this is called 63rd St. Beach, which is a direct reference to where it falls within the street grid, even though 63rd St. becomes Hayes St. west of here. (That name honors Samuel Snowden Hayes, a Civil War–era Chicago politician who was one of the few Democrats then to forcefully oppose slavery.)

- At the east end of the beach, walk to the end of the 400-yard-long breakwater. The views north to the Loop and south along the shore to Rainbow Beach and beyond to Indiana are a fitting reward for the end of your long walk.

- To return, you can take the Metra electric from the 59th St./University of Chicago station or grab a 6 Jackson Park bus.

CONNECTING THE WALKS

From Jackson Park Beach, it is easy to take the underpass west beneath busy S. South Shore Dr. and link up with Walk 2 in Jackson Park. Or walk 1 mile north along the lake to Promontory Point and join Walk 4.

POINTS OF INTEREST

Rainbow Beach Park 3111 E. 77th St., 312-745-1479

Exchange Cafe 7201 S. Exchange Ave., 773-336-8592

South Shore Cultural Center 7059 S. South Shore Dr., 773-256-0149

route summary

1. Start at 67-acre Rainbow Beach Park and walk north along the beach.

2. Cut northwest across the grass to roughly where E. 77th St. would intersect the park.

3. Turn right to head north along S. South Shore Dr.

4. Turn left on 72nd St.; walk two blocks west to S. Exchange St.

5. Turn right on S. Exchange Ave. and walk north.

6. At the intersection of Exchange, E. 71st St., and S. South Shore Dr., cross to the northeast corner and enter the grounds of the South Shore Cultural Center.

7. Exit the South Shore Cultural Center and walk north along S. South Shore Dr.

8. At E. 67th St., follow the sidewalk as it becomes a waterfront path and walk north.

9. At the end of the isthmus, walk back south along the west side.

10. Follow the waterside path west around the north side of E. Marquette Dr.

11. Turn right (north) to cross the Animal Bridge and continue on the wide sidewalk along the water.

12. Cross behind the old Coast Guard Station and continue along the waterfront walk to Jackson Park Beach.

13. At the east end of the beach, walk out to the end of the breakwater.

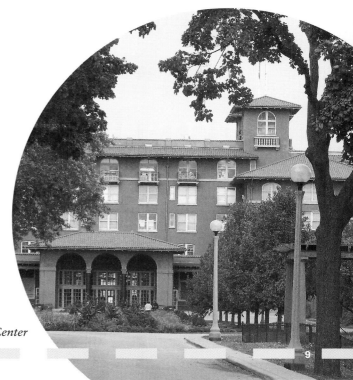

South Shore Cultural Center

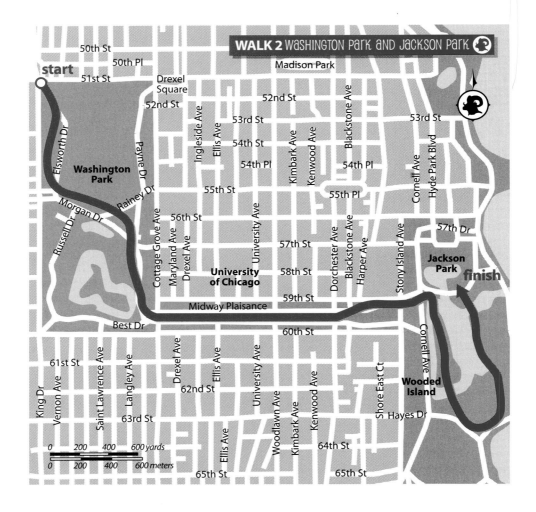

50th St

50th Pl

start

51st St

Madison Park

Drexel Square

52nd St

Ingleside Ave

Ellis Ave

52nd St

53rd St

53rd St

54th St

Payne Dr

Washington Park

Rainey Dr

54th Pl

Kimbark Ave

Kenwood Ave

Blackstone Ave

54th Pl

Cornell Ave

Hyde Park Blvd

55th St

Elsworth Dr

Morgan Dr

Russell Dr

55th Pl

56th St

Cottage Grove Ave

Maryland Ave

Drexel Ave

University Ave

57th St

Dorchester Ave

Blackstone Ave

Harper Ave

Stony Island Ave

57th Dr

Jackson Park

University of Chicago

58th St

finish

59th St

Midway Plaisance

Best Dr

60th St

61st St

King Dr

Vernon Ave

Saint Lawrence Ave

Langley Ave

Drexel Ave

Ellis Ave

University Ave

Woodlawn Ave

Kimbark Ave

Kenwood Ave

Shore East Ct

Cornell Ave

Wooded Island

62nd St

63rd St

Ellis Ave

Hayes Dr

64th St

0   200   400   600 yards

0   200   400   600 meters

65th St

65th St

2 WASHINGTON PARK AND JACKSON PARK: TALES OF THE WHITE CITY

BOUNDARIES: **E. 51st St., Lake Michigan, E. 63rd St., S. King Dr.**
DISTANCE: **4.2 miles (one way)**
PUBLIC TRANSIT: **Green Line El to 51st St.; 3 King Dr. bus**

An area of great renown in the late 1800s, the swath of the South Side that includes Washington and Jackson parks was the destination of millions during the 1893 Columbian Exposition, an early-day world's fair meant to celebrate the anniversary of Columbus's discovery of America (albeit a year late). During its six-month run, more than 27 million people visited an over-the-top assemblage of buildings and attractions designed to celebrate world cultures and the industrial accomplishments of America. (By contrast, Florida's Disney World attracts about 16 million each year.) Much of the architecture was spectacular, and the fair deeply influenced American architecture—and Chicago's in particular. The exposition was known as the "White City" for the brilliant Beaux Arts finish of its buildings, which glowed under thousands of newfangled electric lights.

Today, portions of the fair's grounds survive in Jackson Park, although almost every building is gone, due to their construction of plaster, straw, and other ephemeral materials. The park itself is surprisingly fascinating, with many little-known features, such as natural areas that will have you swearing you're in the middle of remote Wisconsin.

To the west, across the "Midway," Washington Park was built in the 1870s at a time when Chicago's plans for open public spaces were indeed grand. Frederick Law Olmsted, the Michelangelo of 19th-century park designers, produced big plans that literally went up in smoke during the 1871 fire. In those pre-Xerox, hard-drive-backup days, recreating the plans proved to be a challenge, and the park never fulfilled its original promise, though it's quite pretty today. Olmsted went on to design the grounds for the White City and their subsequent conversion into Jackson Park.

● Start in the northwest corner of Washington Park. Across the intersection with E. 55th St, look for the statue of George Washington astride a horse, thrusting his sword into the air. You can see the park through the trees of the park's 30-acre arboretum to the south. Walk south through this half-mile-long patch of trees, from E. 51st St. to E. 55th St. (S. King Dr. is on the west). The huge oaks predate the park; other trees include walnuts, elms, maples and willows.

Where E. 55th St. enters the park, head east across the broad expanse of open grass dotted with softball fields. This open space is the heart of Chicago's bid for the 2016 Olympics, which, if the city wins, will pretty much obliterate the space for a 95,000-seat arena. The scheme calls for the mega-stadium to be mostly removed after the games, but many find this notion incredible. Meantime, the softball players are supplanted by a cricket league on Sunday mornings—although unlike everywhere else in the world where they are played, the games don't last for days (even if it seems that way to spectators).

● At the east end of the fields cross Rainey Dr. and walk south through the formal gardens west of S. Cottage Grove Ave. toward the Classical building home to the DuSable Museum of African American History. Originally a park administration building, this imposing 1910 structure is named for Jean Baptiste Point DuSable, Chicago's first non-native settler, a Haitian man with African heritage. The engrossing museum includes displays documenting everything from slavery to a reconstruction of the City Hall office of Harold Washington, who served as Chicago's first black mayor between 1983 and 1987.

● From the museum, go west and cross Morgan Dr., then follow the curving paths south through what is easily the prettiest section of the park. This is where Olmsted's vision was built, even if it is smaller and less striking than conceived. The irregular lines of the water features and plantings are meant to evoke something you might stumble onto in the woods. What you won't stumble onto is any lingering evidence of the flock of sheep that lived in the park until they were banished in 1920.

Stop at the southeast corner of the park for one of Chicago's great open-air treats, Laredo Taft's *Fountain of Time*. Built to celebrate the peace the United States and Britain had enjoyed since the latter sacked the White House in 1814, the sculpture was completed in 1922. Dozens of enigmatic figures—including the stoic, mustached countenance of University of Chicago prof Taft—are depicted across the 102-foot work's length. Many figures are clearly the worse for the passage of time—as was the entire concrete sculpture until a recent magnificent restoration.

- Walk east from the statue into the Midway Plaisance, the long vista of grass and sidewalks that stretches for almost a mile. In Olmsted's original plan, the Midway was to be a waterway connecting Washington and Jackson parks. Alas, this vision was never carried out. During the Columbian Exposition, the Midway was home to the park's less cultural but wildly more popular attractions such as the world's first Ferris wheel, along with other ancestors of carnival attractions popular in "Midways" today. Millions of visitors took a great interest in Egyptian culture at the Street in Cairo theater, which featured belly dancers doing the hootchie cootchie. Other diversions included the usual bearded ladies, dog-faced boys and the like. Buffalo Bill set up his Wild West Show and reaped millions, to the consternation of exposition backers who didn't want his "populist" act in the White City. Unfortunately, today, the elegant sweep of lawn is broken up by a tacky University of Chicago skating rink. Gridiron fans take note: the "Monsters of the Midway" moniker often (though without good reason) applied to the Chicago Bears was originally a nickname for the University of Chicago's now-defunct football team.

- Cross under the railroad tracks on E. 59th St. and continue east to S. Stony Island Ave. This marks the western edge of the official exposition site, which stretched from here to the lake and north to E. 56th St. and south to E. 67th St.

Fountain of Time, *Washington Park*

- Enter Jackson Park and follow the path that would be an extension of E. 59th St. The wide isthmus with ponds north and south was the location of the Illinois Building. This huge erection had a rather phallic dome and was widely panned. Famed Chicago architect Louis Sullivan (who was responsible for the overall look of the fair but not this building) deemed it a "lewd exhibit of drooling imbecility."

- Continue east until you get to the bridge over the narrow channel of water. To the north is a postcard view of the Museum of Science and Industry, which during the fair was the Fine Arts Building. It escaped the destruction of much of the rest of the White City thanks to its brick sub-structure, which had been specified to protect the displayed works during the fair. It was chosen as the home for a new science museum in the 1920s and the by-then moth-eaten plaster exterior was replaced by the limestone facade you see today.

  The bridge you are standing on is known as the "Clarence Darrow Bridge." The famed attorney lived nearby and often came here to think through his cases, such as his spirited defense of the right to teach evolution in the Scopes Monkey Trial. In order to debunk psychics, Darrow said that after he died he'd return to the bridge to proclaim his existence. Each year on the anniversary of his death (March 13, 10:10 AM) a crowd gathers to recall his life. So far he hasn't shown up, but one would think that, with recent assaults on the theory of evolution, he might put in an appearance.

- Retrace your steps slightly west and then follow the path south across the bridge to the splendor of Wooded Island. This is one of the parts of Jackson Park least changed since the fair, when it was a much-loved refuge from the crowds for strollers and neckers alike. On the northeast corner you'll see the entrance for the suitably serene Japanese Garden, which dates to 1893. From here south the island becomes increasingly wild, and soon you'll find it hard to believe you're in the city at all. Dozens of species attract bird-watchers, while 20 types of fish attract anglers to the ponds. There's even been a boom in beavers: 16 were trapped in 2003 after they started gnawing away on the trees, but a family still lurks in the shadows.

Back Story: The Details are in the Devil

Interest in Jackson Park and the site of the White City has exploded since the publication of Eric Larson's best-selling *Devil in the White City* in 2003. Although it takes some work to discern the links to the Columbian Exposition, on most weekends you'll see people taking organized tours pegged to the book. Larson's genius was to pair the stories of Burnham, Olmsted and others with the exploits of H. H. Holmes (a.k.a. Herman Webster Mudgett), who constructed a hotel of horrors where he literally and fatally boned guests—often fairgoers—and extracted their skeletons for resale to Chicago medical schools. Today the location at W. 63rd St. and S. Wallace Ave. 3 miles west of Jackson Park in the Englewood neighborhood is the site of a post office—which may hold horror for some even now.

● Cross the bridge at the south end of Wooded Island and continue straight on to E. Hayes Dr. To the east in the summer there is often a food trailer near the softball diamond that serves some mighty fine Mexican food, including excellent tamales. Break the cola habit with a tamarind soda.

● Walk east 150 yards along the Hayes Dr. sidewalk until you are standing in front of the statue titled *The Republic*. This large, gold-leafed wonder is *one-third* the size of the original that stood nearby during the fair. It is unofficially known as Bert in honor of Bertha Palmer, the city's premier arts patron in the 19th century. Where you're standing now has seen many changes since 1893. This was the center of the Court of Honor, the elegant assemblage of huge display buildings (Agriculture, Electricity, etc.) around formal canals alive with Venetian gondolas. Nothing of the layout or waterways remain; Olmsted's plan called for the creation of the more naturalistic park after the fair.

● Continue east along Hayes Dr. over the small bridge, then immediately veer north on a narrow trail. This marks the southern extent of the fair's most amazing building, the Brobdingnagian Manufacturers and Liberal Arts Building. In 1893 it was the largest enclosed building ever built and covered 44 acres.

- Follow the path north past the driving range. The terrain rapidly becomes wild prairie, with tall grasses and spectacular wildflowers thriving in the sun all summer long. If Wooded Island across the pond represents a Midwestern forest, this shade-free field recalls the literal oceans of multi-hued prairies that greeted early settlers. Volunteers are working to recreate the native prairie landscape. When you see the first tiny island in the pond, you'll have reached the northern extent of the Manufacturer's Building, nearly 600 yards from its southern extent. The exhibits in the vast hall were mostly display models from various companies. Children's eyes no doubt glazed over at the array of desks from a school furniture manufacturer. Like much of the rest of the White City, the building succumbed to fire in 1894.

- Finish the walk by crossing the bridge over the channel with docks and an outlet to the lake. At Columbia Dr. you can continue north around the east side for a visit of the Museum of Science and Industry.

- Return on the Metra Electric from the 59th St. stop, or take the 6 Jackson Park Express Bus.

CONNECTING THE WALKS

Walk to the east to the lake and south to Jackson Park Beach to link up with the end of Walk 1.

POINTS OF INTEREST

DuSable Museum of African American History www.dusablemuseum.org, 740 E. 56th Pl., 773-947-0600

Museum of Science and Industry www.msichicago.org, W. 57th St. and Lake Shore Dr., 773-684-1414

route summary

1. Start at northwest corner of Washington Park. Walk south from E. 51st St. to E. 55th St. and S. King Dr.

2. Where E. 55th St. enters the park, turn left and head east across the broad expanse of open grass.

3. At the east end of the fields, where E. 55th St. curves into S. Payne Dr., cross Rainey Dr. and walk south through the formal gardens west of S. Cottage Grove Ave. toward the DuSable Museum of African American History

4. From the museum, go west and cross Morgan Dr., then follow the curving paths south.

5. Stop at the southeast corner of the park at Laredo Taft's *Fountain of Time.*

6. Walk east from the statue into the Midway Plaisance.

7. Cross under the railroad tracks on E. 59th St. and continue east to S. Stony Island Ave.

8. Enter Jackson Park and follow the path that would be an extension of E. 59th St.

9. Continue east to the bridge over the narrow channel of water.

10. Retrace your steps slightly west and follow the path south across the bridge to Wooded Island.

11. Cross the bridge at the south end of Wooded Island and continue straight on to E. Hayes Dr.

12. Walk east 150 yards along the Hayes Dr. sidewalk until you are standing in front of *The Republic.*

13. Continue east along Hayes Dr. over the small bridge, then immediately veer north on a narrow trail.

14. Follow the path north past the driving range and on through the reproduced prairie.

15. Finish the walk by crossing the bridge over the channel to Columbia Dr.

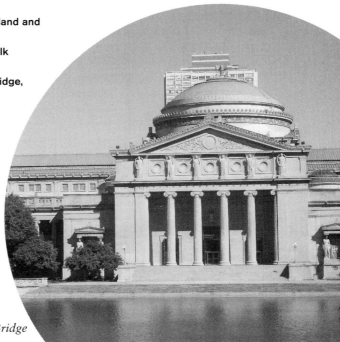

Museum of Science and Industry, from Darrow Bridge

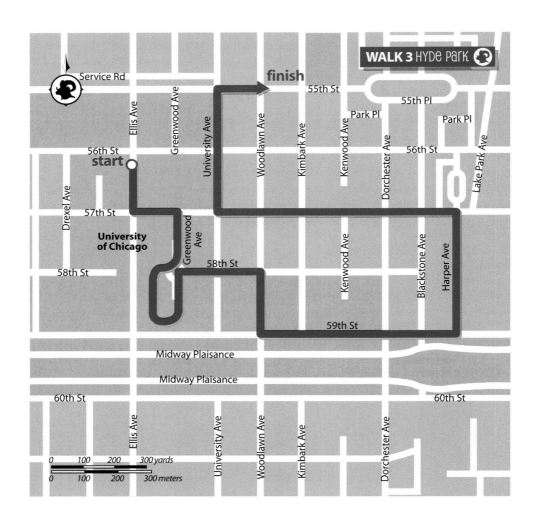

Service Rd

finish

55th St

55th Pl

Park Pl

Park Pl

56th St

56th St

start

57th St

University of Chicago

58th St

58th St

Midway Plaisance

Midway Plaisance

60th St

60th St

Drexel Ave

Ellis Ave

Greenwood Ave

Greenwood Ave

University Ave

Woodlawn Ave

Kimbark Ave

Kenwood Ave

Kenwood Ave

Dorchester Ave

Blackstone Ave

Harper Ave

Lake Park Ave

59th St

Ellis Ave

University Ave

Woodlawn Ave

Kimbark Ave

Dorchester Ave

0   100   200   300 yards

0   100   200   300 meters

3 HYDE PARK: BIG BANGS AND BOOKS AT THE UNIVERSITY OF CHICAGO

BOUNDARIES: **E. 55th St., S. Harper Ave., E. 59th St., S. Ellis Ave.**
DISTANCE: **2½ miles**
PUBLIC TRANSIT: **Metra Electric to 55th-56th-57th stop, 6 Jackson Park Express bus**

Hyde Park's raison d'etre, the University of Chicago, has kept the neighborhood vibrant even as surrounding areas of the South Side have struggled. Perhaps, however, "vibrant" is the wrong word for an institution noted for its deep thinkers. That the U of C has a perennial lock on the Nobel Prize for Economics is a given, but it's also renowned for its programs in theology, literature and dead languages. Physics also makes a bang: this is where the U.S. Manhattan Project had its first crucial success in the quest to build the bomb. Many of the University's buildings are done up in classic Gothic designs featuring rich carvings, making it an endlessly engrossing place for a stroll. Bookstores way outnumber bars in Hyde Park; bibliophiles may wish to bring a sturdy backpack, drinkers a six-pack.

- **Start the tour of the University of Chicago and Hyde Park with a bang just south of the corner of E. 56th St. and S. Ellis Ave. On the east side of the street, look for the large bronze sculpture that looks like a skull combined with a mushroom cloud. This is *Nuclear Energy*, the 1967 work that commemorates the start of the nuclear age when Enrico Fermi and his colleagues achieved their first self-sustaining atomic reaction at 3:53 PM on Dec. 2, 1942. Back then this was the site of the school's abandoned Stagg Field, and the scientists had their labs under the stands—despite a few hand-wringers who thought the test might take out most of Hyde Park. One later said: "We had known we were about to unlock a giant; still, we could not escape an eerie feeling when we knew we had actually done it." Today there are dorms on the site, so if some of the students seem to have a healthy glow . . .**

- **Continue south on S. Ellis Ave. and turn east on E. 57th St. The building on the northeast corner is the Regenstein Library, a 1970 Brutalist expression in concrete by Walter Netsch (the man responsible for much of the University of Illinois at Chicago campus that was later torn down to popular acclaim). Many critics wish** another try at nuclear energy would go wrong and obliterate this atrocity, although the bunker-like windows would probably repel the blast.

- Immediately across from the library entrance, pass south through Cobb Gate. This 1900 fantasy of carved limestone features a series of gargoyles trying to claw their way to the top, a tableau some say represents undergrads. Certainly many do struggle with the U of C's academic rigor, although many more thrive in the other-worldly nature of the campus where some degrees aren't completed even after a decade or more of intellectual pursuit. (The *only* time the U of C can be compared to *Animal House* is when John Belushi laments: "Seven years of college down the drain.")

- Continue on until you are in the aesthetic heart of campus, the Main Quadrangle. The shady open space features benches you may not want to leave, huge shade trees and students sprawled on the grass thinking big thoughts (or how to tell their parents they'll need an eighth year of tuition). Spin around and take in this collection of academic buildings, which date from a span of decades beginning in the 1890s. This is college Gothic architecture at its most flamboyant. Carved details relating to areas of thought and study abound. Look for the George Herbert Jones Laboratory building in the northwest corner. In 1942, researchers first isolated plutonium here. Room 405 was where the work took place; the federal government spent years in the 1980s removing radioactive waste.

- From the center of the quad, walk southwest and pass between Cobb Hall (1892) and Bond Chapel. The latter is an ecclesiastic gem and features a lute player carved into the cornice. The south façade of the chapel fronts the Classics Quadrangle. This intimate space is surrounded by ornately detailed buildings. They are (going clockwise from Bond Chapel): Frederick Haskell Hall (1896), Wiebolt Hall (1928), the Classics Building (1915) and Cobb Hall. Among the myriad details, look for famous authors on Wiebolt and—fittingly—characters from Aesop's Fables on Classics.

- Exit the quad through the arch at the southeast corner and turn north in front of the twin-towered, iconic William Rainey Harper Memorial Library (1912) and return to the center of the main quad.

- Turn east and cross S. University Ave. Immediately across from each other on E. 58th St. are two diversions that might throw a monkeywrench into your timetable. On the north side, the Chicago Theological Seminary is home to the Seminary Co-op Bookstore, which has a seemingly endless selection of academic titles in its warren-like cellar location. Where else can you get a copy of the classic account of the Peloponnesian War by Thucydides (and wouldn't he be chuffed to know it was still in print?). On the south side of 58th is the Oriental Institute, the university's own antiquities museum. This is where the real Indiana Jones hung out; inside, treasures from Mesopotamia and Egypt include Assyrian carvings from the time of King Sargon II. Large photos show these ancient sites today, such as the lonely, green fields of Anatolia that were once the domain of the Hittites.

- Continue east on E. 58th St. to the northeast corner with S. Woodlawn Ave. If you see someone with round "artsy" glasses genuflecting, it's probably another architect on pilgrimage to Robie House, one of Frank Lloyd Wright's finest works. Built in 1909, its long horizontal lines and intricate modern detailing immediately made its neighbors look like a bunch of frumps. Tours of the artful interior are worthwhile.

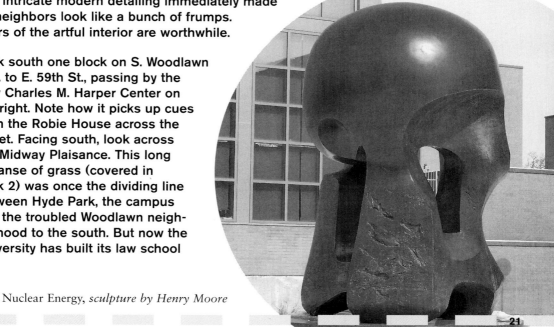

- Walk south one block on S. Woodlawn Ave. to E. 59th St., passing by the new Charles M. Harper Center on the right. Note how it picks up cues from the Robie House across the street. Facing south, look across the Midway Plaisance. This long expanse of grass (covered in Walk 2) was once the dividing line between Hyde Park, the campus and the troubled Woodlawn neighborhood to the south. But now the University has built its law school

Nuclear Energy, *sculpture by Henry Moore*

south of the Midway and the neighborhood is on the rise. Facing north, to your left is the soaring tower of Rockefeller Memorial Chapel (1928). Dozens of religious sculptures can be found inside and out.

● Walk a half block east on E. 59th St. and enter Ida Noyes Hall. Built in 1916, the detailed Tudor Revival interior is a riot of richly carved wood. Head up to the third floor to the theater to see the 1918 mural *The Masque of Youth*, an allegorical representation of campus life. The hall was built at a time when women students were banned from many of the common areas of campus with the exception of this one. For insight to campus life today, go down to The Pub, the casual basement student bar featuring lots of decent beer and cheap pizza. It's supposedly a private club but membership comes easy to those with charm.

● Exit Noyes Hall and continue east on E. 59th St. past various imposing school buildings. Just before the railroad viaduct turn north on S. Harper Ave. The 5700 and 5800 blocks here are the site of the Rosalie Villas, one of Chicago's first planned developments. A female entrepreneur, Rosalie Buckingham, subdivided the land and hired Solon S. Beman, the architect of Pullman (see Walk 7) to work his intricate magic here. Considering that most of the houses date from the late 1880s, the street is surprisingly intact, having resisted the ravages of time and the varying priorities of owners. (It's said locally that Nobel Laureates have the worst-maintained houses as they're too busy being brilliant to have time to trim the shrubs. Given that the U of C has had 81 laureates, that's a lot of deferred maintenance.) Among the houses to look for: 5810, which bucks the wood and shingle motif of the street; 5736, a lavish multi-porched fantasy that predates the rest of the block, and 5732, a fantasy (or nightmare) in purple that reflects the street's funky charm.

● Stop at E. 57th St. On the southeast corner is Powell's Used Bookstore, the first of many places for book-lovers on this leafy yet popular commercial strip.

● Walk west on E. 57th St., and don't be surprised if you see one of the aforementioned Nobel Laureates shambling along eating an ice cream cone. At 1448, the O'Gara & Wilson bookshop, lethargic ceiling fans gently rustle the dust on the tall shelves of ancient and rare volumes. Farther up past S. Kenwood Ave, Medici Bakery is good for a snack. Next door, the otherwise un-noteworthy University Market has a classic

Hyde Park bulletin board out front. This is the place to find a flyer advertising a tutor in classical languages or a fencing school for children. At the corner of S. Kimbark Ave., 57th Street Books is a basement labyrinth with a varied and mainstream selection plus frequent author events.

- At S. University Ave., turn north and enter the building on the left, Bartlett Hall. Built as a gymnasium in 1902, it features the usual over-the-top carving outside and some artistic surprises inside. On the second floor, you can't miss the long mural of medieval athletic tournaments. Stoic knights, pensive trumpeters and doleful queens are but some of the features of this creation that cries out for a little animation *á la* Terry Gilliam. Note the inscription over the door that reads in part: "To the advancement of Physical Education and the Glory of Manly Sports . . . "

- Walk north on S. University Ave. Turn east on E. 55th St. and go almost to the northwest corner with S. Woodlawn Ave. By now you're probably thirsty and no Hyde Park/ U of C visit is complete without a stop at the Woodlawn Tap (a.k.a. Jimmy's), a perfectly idiosyncratic bar for the community. Bartenders pick the music and serve up $2.50 cheeseburgers on small paper plates. The books behind the bar are weighty reference tomes for sorting out philosophical debates. Just watch yourself on the way out, as the step down is a killer and drunk patrons only return after a visit to the ER.

- Walk east to the Metra Electric to the 55th-56th-57th stop and 6 Jackson Park Express bus, or take the 55 55th St. bus west to the Garfield stops on the El Green and Red lines.

POINTS OF INTEREST

University of Chicago www.uchicago.edu, 801 S. Ellis Ave., 773-702-1234

Robie House www.wrightplus.org, 5757 S. Woodlawn Ave., 708-848-1976

Seminary Co-op Bookstore 5757 S. University Ave., 773-752-4381

Oriental Institute 1155 E. 58th St., 773-702-9514

The Pub Ida Noyes Hall, 1212 E. 59th St., 773-702-9737

Powell's Used Bookstore 1501 E. 57th St., 773-955-7780

O'Gara & Wilson 1448 E. 57th St., 773-363-0993

University Market 1323 E. 57th St., 773-363-0070

57th Street Books 1301 E. 57th St., 773-684-1300

Woodlawn Tap 1172 E. 55th St., 773-643-5516

route summary

1. Start the tour of the University of Chicago and Hyde Park just south of the corner of E. 56th St. and S. Ellis Ave.
2. Go south on S. Ellis Ave. and turn left on E. 57th St.
3. Immediately across from the Regenstein Library entrance, pass south through Cobb Gate.
4. Continue to the Main Quadrangle.
5. From the center of the quad, walk southwest and pass between Cobb Hall and Bond Chapel.
6. Exit the quad through the arch at the southeast corner and turn north in front of the William Rainey Harper Memorial Library and return to the center of the main quad.
7. Turn right and cross S. University Ave. heading east.
8. Continue east on E. 58th St. to the northeast corner with S. Woodlawn Ave.
9. Turn right and walk south one block on S. Woodlawn Ave. to E. 59th St.
10. Turn left and walk a half block east on E. 59th St.; enter Ida Noyes Hall.
11. Exit Noyes Hall and continue east on E. 59th St.
12. Just before the railroad viaduct turn north on S. Harper Ave.
13. Walk west on E. 57th St.
14. At S. University Ave., turn right and enter the building on the left, Bartlett Hall.
15. Walk north on S. University Ave.
16. Turn right on E. 55th St. and go to the northwest corner with S. Woodlawn Ave.

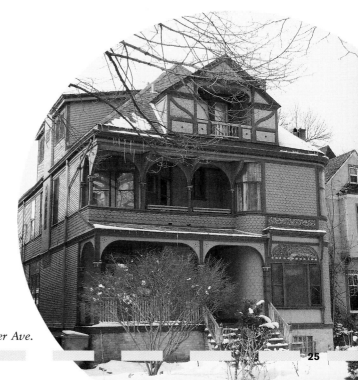

Victorian house at 5736 S. Harper Ave.

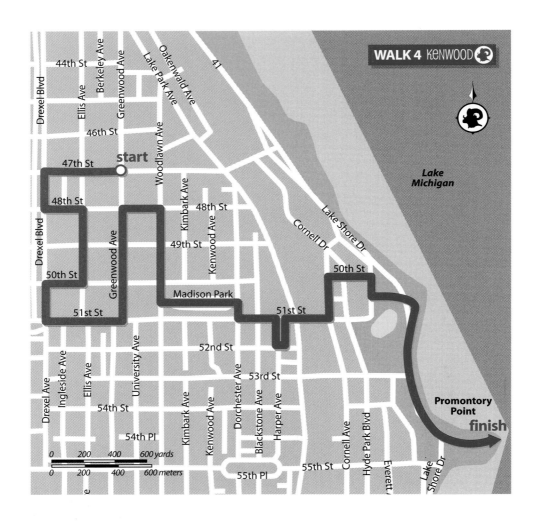

44th St

Drexel Blvd

Berkeley Ave

Ellis Ave

Greenwood Ave

Lake Park Ave

Oakenwald Ave

41

Lake Michigan

46th St

47th St

start

Woodlawn Ave

48th St

Drexel Blvd

Greenwood Ave

Kimbark Ave

48th St

Kenwood Ave

Cornell Dr

Lake Shore Dr

49th St

50th St

50th St

Madison Park

51st St

51st St

52nd St

Drexel Ave

Ingleside Ave

Ellis Ave

University Ave

Kimbark Ave

53rd St

Kenwood Ave

Dorchester Ave

Blackstone Ave

Harper Ave

54th St

Promontory Point

finish

54th Pl

Cornell Ave

Hyde Park Blvd

Everett

Lake Shore Dr

55th St

55th Pl

0   200   400   600 yards

0   200   400   600 meters

4 KENWOOD: BLACK AND WHITE SO HEAD ON OVER

BOUNDARIES: E. 47th St., Lake Michigan, E. 51st St., S. Drexel Blvd.
DISTANCE: 4 miles
PUBLIC TRANSIT: Metra Electric to 47th stop, 3 Jackson Park Express bus, 47 47th St. bus from Green and Red Line El 47th St. stops

Kenwood became fashionable in the late 1800s when rich Chicagoans fled the industrialization and prostitution of Prairie Ave. to the north (see Walk 13). Vast mansions were built over a period of several decades and the neighborhood was the home of many European Jews. After World War II, the same demographic changes that caused upheaval across the South Side were felt here. But owing to their wealth and determination to preserve their neighborhood, residents fought against panic selling and other changes. One key weapon: constant zoning challenges to prevent large mansions from being chopped up into rooming houses, an alteration that had doomed other upscale neighborhoods. Concurrently, many middle class and wealthy African-Americans were moving into Kenwood. In fact many sardonically said the local motto should be: "Black and white united to keep out the poor." As you walk the mannered streets today enjoying the lush gardens and renovated mansions, you'll appreciate both the truth in the phrase and the reality.

● Start at the northwest corner of E. 47th St. and S. Greenwood Ave. The Hidden Pearl Art Cafe is just the place to gather your bearings for Kenwood. It's the caffeinated front end of the renowned Little Black Pearl Art and Design Center, which is a thriving non-profit offering programs to South Side kids in some of the most-troubled African-American neighborhoods. While you imbibe, check out the many amazing works for sale and chat with a few of the artists.

● Head two blocks west to the southeast corner of S. Drexel Blvd. and E. 47th St. The mannered 1920s Sutherland Hotel has been restored and offers affordable housing behind its tidy brick façade. But the big noise here was in the 1950s and 1960s when the likes of Dizzy Gillespie, Louis Armstrong, and John Coltrane regularly performed. Efforts are underway to have top-notch jazz played here again. Such energies could benefit all of E. 47th St., which in its 1920s heyday was the commercial heart of Black Chicago.

- Walk one block south on S. Drexel Blvd. Named for an early Chicago banker, Drexel Blvd. is a key link in the city's extensive system of boulevards: extra-wide, lushly landscaped streets joining major parks that were built in the late 1800s (for more see Walk 29).

- Turn east on E. 48th St. and go to the intersection with S. Ellis Ave. Stop here for a minute to soak up the buildings around you and you'll immediately understand why many in the know consider Kenwood the most attractive neighborhood in the city. The impressive houses around you date from the late 19th and early 20th centuries and are exquisitely detailed with features like turrets, colonnades and more.

- Stroll south along S. Ellis Ave. Houses of note here include: No. 4800, with grand double turrets (1898). No. 4832 has a vast wrap-around porch. See if you can make friends here so you can enjoy a gin and tonic from its shady confines. At 4848, look for the letter *S* in the terra-cotta details in honor of the owner, mega-meatpacker Gustavus Swift (1898). 4901 is an over-the-top limestone confection that was home to Julius Rosenwald, the head of Sears when it was conquering the United States (1903). At 4928, note the evil squirrels decorating corners of the deck (1901).

- Walk one block west on E. 50th St. On the northeast corner with S. Drexel Blvd. is the imposing colonnaded headquarters of Jesse Jackson's Operation Push. Look across Drexel and slightly north to 4938, an 1890 French medieval fantasy right out of the Loire Valley. After a checkered middle age during which it was among other things a flophouse for hippies, it's now upscale condos.

- Head south on S. Drexel Blvd. one block to E. Hyde Park Blvd. Look across the intersection to where the boulevard makes a 90-degree turn west to meet up with Washington Park, and you'll see Drexel Fountain, renovated so that it looks better than when it was new in 1880.

- Walk one block east on E. Hyde Park Blvd. (a.k.a. E. 51st St.) and stop at the north-west corner of S. Ellis Ave. Long derelict, the mansion here was once home to the family of Bobby Franks, the boy who was kidnapped and murdered just up the block on E. 50th St. by Nathan Leopold and Richard Loeb in 1924. The crime was a sensa-tion owing to the wealth of the perps and their stunning defense by Clarence Darrow (he saved them from hanging). Plays based on the crime are regularly performed and the case formed the basis of Hitchcock's *Rope*, which features Jimmy Stewart chewing the carpet for the ages.

- One more block east on Hyde Park Blvd., stop at the northwest corner of S. Greenwood Ave. Spend too much time peering at the evergreen hedge and wrought-iron fencing of the house set back from Greenwood and a stern dude in shades may emerge from an unmarked sedan and ask you your business. Answer that you're just checking out the home of Barack Obama, whose run for president has put this house on the map. The Obama manse is a comfortable wood-trimmed house typical of this upscale neighborhood. But it has one difference: an extra-wide lot, thanks to Obama's purchase of a swatch of the vacant-but-landscaped corner lot from Chicago power-broker Tony Rezko, whose questionable political activities made headlines. Note that Obama's neighbor across the street is the K. A. M. Isaiah Israel Temple, the oldest synagogue in Chicago.

- Perambulate north on S. Greenwood Ave. Another lovely Kenwood street, Greenwood's highlights include: 4840, a Tudor dream with rich carvings including lions and angels (1902), and 4835, which is not an electrical substation but rather an imposing modern brick house.

- Turn east on E. 48th St., walk one block east to S. Woodlawn Ave., and turn south. One of Kenwood's oldest houses (1873) is at 4812. You can still see how the wealthy traveled back then: first the horse was tied up to the horse ring held by an iron fist, and then the passengers alighted from the carriage, avoiding any nastiness in the gutter by using the stone steps at the curb. Farther south at the northeast corner with E. 49th St.

The home of Barack Obama, Kenwood

you'll see a rather large and garish modern mansion. It was home to Nation of Islam founder Elijah Muhammad and is now occupied by his successor, Louis Farrakhan. Those tidy guys you see in bow ties are the Fruits of Islam, the security force. At 4944, you could have once had a pounding of a different kind: the vast Tudor mansion was owned by Muhammad Ali.

- Just south of E. 50th St. turn east into Madison Park, a collection of houses and apartments on a private road (prominently posted for "10 M.P.H."). The quarter-mile long enclave has houses in a variety of 20th-century styles. Overhead, you'll likely hear the squawk of the local parakeets. Yes, you heard that right, Kenwood and Hyde Park are home to several flocks of parakeets descended from birds that literally flew the coop from their owners in the lakefront high-rises. Look for a flash of green as they zip past.

- At S. Dorchester Ave. turn north and walk about 100 feet. The squat walls on the west side of the street reveal little of what lies inside their bunker-like facades: large, light-filled apartments with glass walls facing central courtyards. A sign marks the unit once owned by Bill Veeck, the legendary baseball promoter who owned the White Sox in 1979 when "Disco Demolition Night" turned into a riot. He was famous for keeping his home phone number listed in the phone book. He said at the time he didn't mind drunks calling at 2 AM because from time to time it was somebody with a good idea.

- Walk the bases south to E. Hyde Park Blvd. and turn east until you get to S. Harper Ave. and then walk another block south. The New Checkerboard Lounge is the gussied-up successor to the legendary blues club that closed in 2003. Although it lacks the grit of the original, that's probably a good thing, as the 43rd St. location was condemned by the city.

- Back on Hyde Park Blvd. jive your way east under the tracks and turn one block north on S. Cornell Ave. You're right in the thicket of some startlingly tall apartment buildings that rose just prior to the stock market crash in 1929. The Narragansett Apartments at 1640 E. 50th St. and the Powhatan Apartments at 1648 are some of the most embellished buildings in Chicago. On the former look for elephants gazing down from the façade. On the latter—the real star of the bunch—notice how Native American themes have been used as inspiration for Art Deco designs that extend from the exterior limestone to the lavish public spaces. The restored lobby is alive with polychromatic murals by Charles Morgan, who used a secret process to give the panels an inner luminosity.

- Cross east into Harold Washington Park. It's named for the city's first African-American mayor, a Hyde Park resident whose apartment overlooked this patch of public space when it had the imaginative name of East End Park. Home to several flocks of feral parakeets, the park got a major injection of buzz in 2007 when the 1974 sculpture *Ecstasy* (look at the shape and the spurting fountains, you'll get it) was restored along with its surrounding reflecting pool. The latter has a booth renting model yachts that young skippers can set sail across the broad waters in temperate months.

- Take the Hyde Park Blvd. pedestrian bridge over S. Lake Shore Dr. to the lakefront and follow the shore south to where it curves out into the lake to form Promontory Point. Thanks to under-engineering back in the day, the city's seawall on Lake Michigan is crumbling. Thanks to Chicago's clout in Congress, zillions of federal tax dollars are flowing in to build new, grander seawalls. However, this being Chicago, there are several catches: the new walls are much bigger and much less attractive than the old walls (read: ugly). Further, many of the old walls were made out of rough-cut limestone, which had a definite charm. But despite provisions in the federal funds to use limestone where appropriate, the various local government agencies decided to use concrete—an affront to locals but not a surprise to any fan of *The Sopranos* who has seen the role concrete can play in local politics. After years of fighting, the locals—with the help of Sen. Obama—won the fight. As you see all the people enjoying this plot of green with its sweeping views and offbeat character, you'll know that for once the good guys won. Previous battles by the always-activist locals included protests over anti-aircraft missiles that were located here during the Cold War and the designation in the late 1960s of an official bongo-drum playing area.

- Walk west for the Metra Electric from the 55th-56th-57th station; 6 Jackson Park bus.

CONNECTING THE WALKS

You can extend your walk south along the lake by walking one mile past the narrow 57th St. Beach and joining up with Walk 1 at Jackson Park Beach. Going north, you can join Walk 5 where it ends at the Hyde Park Blvd. pedestrian bridge.

POINTS OF INTEREST

Hidden Pearl Art Cafe 1060 E. 47th St., 773-285-1211

New Checkerboard Lounge 5201 S. Harper Ct., 773-684-1472

ROUTE SUMMARY

1.   Start at the northwest corner of E. 47th St. and S. Greenwood Ave.

2.   Head two blocks west on E. 47th St. to the southeast corner of S. Drexel Blvd.

3.   Turn left and walk one block south on S. Drexel Blvd.

4.   Turn left on E. 48th St. and go east to the intersection with S. Ellis Ave.

5.   Turn right and walk south along S. Ellis Ave.

6.   Turn right on E. 50th St. and walk one block west.

7.   Turn left on S. Drexel Blvd and walk one block to E. Hyde Park Blvd. (a.k.a. E. 51st St.).

8.   Turn left and walk two blocks east on E. Hyde Park Blvd.

9.   Turn left and walk north on S. Greenwood Ave.

10.   Turn right on E. 48th St. and walk one block east.

11.   Turn right on S. Woodlawn Ave.

12.   Just south of E. 50th St. turn left into Madison Park.

13.   At S. Dorchester Ave. turn left and walk about 100 feet.

14.   Walk south to E. Hyde Park Blvd.

15.   Go east until you get to S. Harper Ave. turn right, and then walk another block south.

16.   Back on Hyde Park Blvd. go east under the tracks and turn left; go one block north on S. Cornell Ave.

17.   Turn right on E. 50th St.

18.   Cross east into Harold Washington Park.

19.   Take the Hyde Park Blvd. pedestrian bridge over S. Lake Shore Dr. to the lakefront and follow the shore south to where it curves out into the lake to form Promontory Point.

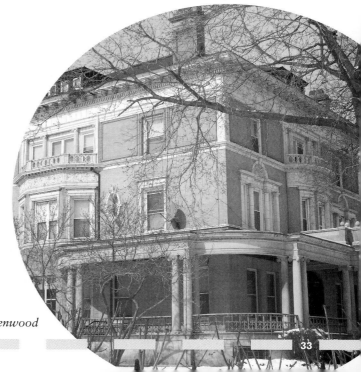

4848 S. Ellis Ave., Kenwood

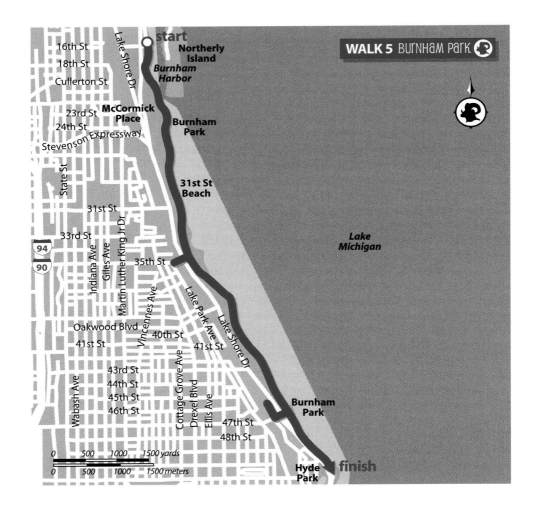

start

Northerly
Island

*Burnham
Harbor*

16th St

18th St

Cullerton St

Lake Shore Dr

**McCormick
Place**

23rd St

24th St

Stevenson Expressway

**Burnham
Park**

State St

**31st St
Beach**

31st St

33rd St

Indiana Ave

Giles Ave

Martin Luther King Jr Dr

94

90

35th St

Vincennes Ave

Lake Park Ave

Lake Shore Dr

*Lake
Michigan*

Oakwood Blvd

40th St

41st St

Cottage Grove Ave

Drexel Blvd

Ellis Ave

41st St

43rd St

44th St

45th St

46th St

Wabash Ave

47th St

48th St

**Burnham
Park**

0   500   1000   1500 yards

0   500   1000   1500 meters

**Hyde
Park**

finish

5   BurNham Park: Placid Balm for a Turbulent Past

BOUNDARIES: **Soldier Field, Lake Michigan, Hyde Park Blvd., Metra Electric tracks**
DISTANCE: **5½ miles**
PUBLIC TRANSIT: **12 Roosevelt bus, 146 Inner Drive/Michigan Express bus**

Seemingly serene, this long and linear lakefront walk through Burnham Park covers a lot of ground that's been contentious, embarrassing or simply notorious in the city's past. The park is named after Chicago's great planner Daniel Burnham, who envisioned a lakefront park on the South Side as early as the 1890s. However, the inevitable delays meant that the six-mile long park linking Grant and Jackson parks didn't really come to fruition until the 1920s and 1930s. Before then the lakefront was swampy and dotted with small beaches. Even when the park was first complete, however, access was hampered by the existing Illinois Central railroad tracks and South Lake Shore Drive, which was completed as part of the park. In fact access is still a problem, and much of the park south of McCormick Place is very quiet. A smattering of joggers, anglers, bike-riders and walkers enjoy the solitude.

● Start near Burnham Harbor in the grassy verge east of S. Museum Campus Dr. and just north of E. Waldron Dr. You are literally in the shadow of Soldier Field, the stadium opened in the 1920s for huge events drawing more than 100,000. In a typical tale, its cost ran more than triple its budget and included a fair amount of cash kickbacks to politicians at the time. In its original form the stadium was so vast that it had to be shrunk several times to make it appropriate for football. The Bears moved here in 1971, and for the next two decades had mediocre success, excepting the 1985 Super Bowl season. Modeled after an imagined Roman stadium of the *Ben-Hur* ilk, Soldier Field (named in honor of World War I servicemen) was a classical icon for the thousands driving past daily on Lake Shore Dr.

This changed in 2001 when it was closed for the $600 million reconstruction you see now. Many think it is the result of an architect with a crash fantasy for alien spaceships, and indeed it's hard to imagine a more egregious sacking of what had been a National Historic Landmark (the National Park Service stripped its designation when it saw the results). If the spaceship-blue growth above the mannered Doric columns on the east side looks odd, check out the west side, where it looks like a science-fiction bun squashing a feeble alien patty. Of course Mayor Daley's fingerprints are all over this: he wanted a new stadium and he got a new stadium, critics be damned. (Not unlike what happened with old Meigs Field across the harbor; see Walk 6.)

● Notice the old Roman column standing next to the Lakefront Trail and behind the Gold Star Families Memorial (which honors those who have lost a relative during war). If the column looks tired, it's not just from the ravages of Chicago weather; the column is more than 2,000 years old, and traveled to Chicago from Ostia, the ancient Roman port. The column was a gift from Benito Mussolini—a man whose actions helped grow the number of Gold Star families.

This entire area was the site of the 1933 Century of Progress world's fair, a landmark event for Chicago that rivals the 1893 Columbian Exposition in importance to the city. Italian aviator Italo Balbo led a flight of seaplanes that touched down in the harbor as part of the exhibition. In its exuberant response, the city renamed 7th St. for Balbo, and the Italian dictator sent the column you see here in thanks. Check out the inscription facing away from the trail, which includes: "Fascist Italy by command of Benito Mussolini presents to Chicago . . . in the eleventh year of the Fascist era." Oops. Besides the whole fascism thing not working out because of World War II, Balbo perished in the war after he was shot down by his own troops.

● Follow the sinuous lakefront path south for about half a mile until you are standing behind McCormick Place. Dubbed the "mistake on the lake" and other pejoratives, the vast cinder-colored slab known as the Lakeside Center replaced a previous fire-proof McCormick Place that burnt down in 1967. The location is the result of clout-heavy lobbying on the part of the *Chicago Tribune*, which dumped on the dreams of those who wanted the lakefront "forever open, clear and free" in order to have a prominent convention center built in the name of its eccentric owner, Col. Robert McCormick. Proposals keep surfacing to install a municipal casino in the building, a doomed project which may be a fitting tribute to the colonel, who fought to keep the country out of World War II.

Just south of the Lakeside Center, look for three acres of prairie flowers and grasses that serve as a sanctuary for migratory birds. There's a small viewing area.

● Walk south along the lake for another half mile. This portion of Burnham Park could not be blander, and maybe that is the idea. Amidst the featureless grass and smattering of juvenile trees is the legacy of one of Chicago's worst moments. On July 27, 1919, an African-American teenager drifted from the 27th St. Beach down to the 29th St. Beach and tried to exit the water. But there was one problem; he had started at a black beach and ended up at a white beach. In their outrage at this violation, the whites at 29th stoned the youth and he drowned. What followed was four days of savage race rioting on the South Side, which killed 40, injured over 500 and destroyed over 1,000 homes by fire. Much of the carnage was in the checkerboard of white and black neighborhoods west of the lake in Bridgeport. Among the white gangs most involved was the Hamburg Athletic Club, a tough bunch that included Richard J. Daley, father of the current mayor and legendary mayor in his own right. Today all traces of the beaches have been erased but the scars on race relations in the city remain.

● Another half mile brings you to the typically placid 31st St. Beach. This entire area of the park has been enjoying a lot of investment in recent years. Near the parking lots south of the bridge, there's a playground named for Bill Berry, a forceful leader of the local Urban League beginning in the 1950s, who fought hard to desegregate the city. In his first days in Chicago, he stood outside skyscrapers in the Loop and counted the number of blacks he saw entering or leaving. He usually didn't get above zero.

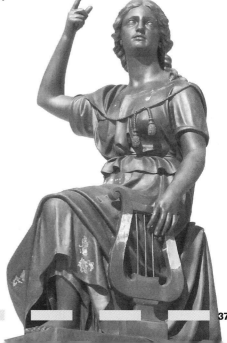

Detail, Stephen A. Douglas tomb and memorial

● Walk across the picnic areas to the skateboard park near the northbound off-ramp from Lake Shore Dr. Half-pipes and more are popular at this lavish study in concrete.

● Continue for another 400 yards south and cross the double pedestrian bridge over S. Lake Shore Dr. and the railroad tracks. From the end of E. 35th St. it's just a few yards to the entrance to the Stephen A. Douglas Tomb and Memorial. A statue of the diminutive Douglas (he was 5'4") sits atop a nearly 100-foot-tall column. A powerful senator from Illinois in the 1850s, he was generally pro-slavery but not quite enough for his Democratic Party. The southern states refused to support him in the 1860 election, which went to the anti-slavery Republican Abraham Lincoln. The pair had a renowned series of debates during their race for a Senate seat in 1858 in which Douglas used the same racist arguments that some politicians try to invoke today. The rather over-wrought memorial is on this spot because like any good Chicago politician, Douglas had a real estate empire based here. Across 35th, the Cardinal Meyer Center holds the offices of the Archdiocese of Chicago and dates from the Civil War, when it was a hospital.

● Cross back over the bridge, but pause while you are over the train tracks. This was once the main line of the Illinois Central Railroad, route of the famed City of New Orleans and a direct link to the bayous and cotton fields of the Deep South. It was the main line for the Great Migration (see the sidebar on page 39).

● Resume your southward trek through Burnham Park. The stretch for about a mile south of the 35th St. pedestrian bridge is especially desolate. Here you'll not only find a fair bit of serenity but also a few folks resolutely fishing throughout the year. From spring to fall, perch, various bass, carp and generic panfish are easily hooked.

● At the E. 47th St. exit off S. Lake Shore Dr., walk west from the park and under the drive to the Burnham Prairie Path. This ever-expanding enclosed area is a new and welcome feature to the otherwise somewhat monotonous grass and trees of the greater park. Boardwalks and trails meander through a symphony of wildflowers and native plants. There's something in bloom most times outside of winter, and you may even catch a flash of color in the air—parts are designed as butterfly gardens.

Back Story: The Great Migration

In 1910 there were 44,000 black people living in Chicago. Ten years later the total was 110,000. A combination of African-American boosters looking to bolster the clout of their community and white business owners looking for cheap, union-busting labor spread the word throughout the South that Chicago was a worker's paradise. Of course it wasn't, but for scores of people, the opportunities in the North outweighed the ongoing oppression in places like Mississippi and Louisiana. This huge shift of population came to be called the Great Migration. Blacks initially settled in South Side neighborhoods that were close to the Illinois Central tracks, the main route used by the new residents. And it wasn't a one-way conduit either on their trek north. Trains heading south carried copies of African-American newspapers like the *Chicago Defender* that carried positive stories about Chicago and encouraged southern blacks to challenge the racism and prejudice of the South. At every stop Pullman porters (who were universally black) distributed the news to a waiting audience.

● **Back in Burnham Park it is a little over half a mile south to the Hyde Park Blvd. pedestrian bridge that will take you into Hyde Park.**

● **Walk west into Hyde Park for the Metra Electric from the 55th-56th-57th station; 6 Jackson Park bus.**

Connecting the Walks

You can extend your walk south by joining Walk 4 at the pedestrian bridge. In the north you can link up with Walk 6, which covers the Museum Campus and Grant Park.

POINTS OF INTEREST

Stephen A. Douglas Tomb and Memorial 800 E. 35th St., 312-744-6630

Burnham Park at the foot of E. 35th St.

ROUTE SUMMARY

1. Start near Burnham Harbor east of S. Museum Campus Dr. and just north of E. Waldron Dr.
2. Follow the lakefront path south for about half a mile until you are standing behind McCormick Place.
3. Walk south along the lake for one mile to 31st St. Beach.
4. Walk across the picnic areas to the skateboard park near the northbound off-ramp from Lake Shore Dr.
5. Continue for another 400 yards south and cross the double pedestrian bridge over S. Lake Shore Dr. and the railroad tracks. From the end of E. 35th St. walk to the Stephen A. Douglas Tomb and Memorial.
6. Cross back over the bridge.
7. Continue south through Burnham Park.
8. At the E. 47th St. exit off S. Lake Shore Dr., walk west from the park and under the drive to the Burnham Prairie Path.
9. Return to the lake path in Burnham Park and walk south to the Hyde Park Blvd. pedestrian bridge.

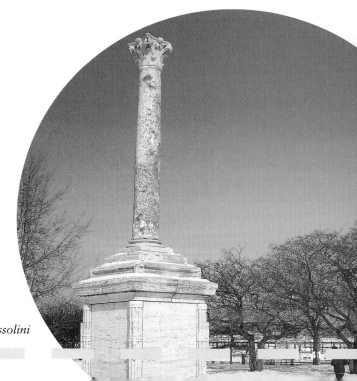

Balbo memorial, with inscription by Mussolini

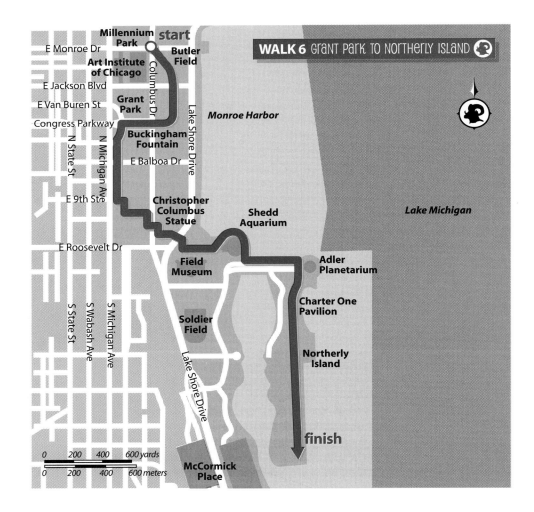

Millennium Park

start

E Monroe Dr

Art Institute of Chicago

E Jackson Blvd

E Van Buren St

Congress Parkway

N State St

N Michigan Ave

Grant Park

Buckingham Fountain

E Balboa Dr

E 9th St

E Roosevelt Dr

S State St

S Wabash Ave

S Michigan Ave

Butler Field

Columbus Dr

Lake Shore Drive

Monroe Harbor

WALK 6 Grant Park to Northerly Island

Christopher Columbus Statue

Field Museum

Soldier Field

Lake Shore Drive

Shedd Aquarium

Adler Planetarium

Charter One Pavilion

Northerly Island

Lake Michigan

finish

McCormick Place

0   200   400   600 yards

0   200   400   600 meters

6 GranT Park To NorTHerly IslanD: FounTains, MuseuMs anD BeacHes

BOUNDARIES: E. Monroe St., Lake Michigan, Northerly Island, S. Michigan Ave.
DISTANCE: 3½ miles
PUBLIC TRANSIT: Numerous El and bus lines just west

Grant Park has often been called Chicago's front yard, and in its present guise it is a show-piece. But that wasn't always the case. In the late 1800s it was a swampy wasteland littered with debris from the fire and shacks filled with bums. Meanwhile, developers who understood its potential began planning numerous developments there. Into the midst of this mess came Montgomery Ward, who was angered at what he saw from his office at 6 N. Michigan Ave. and fought to preserve, as the line in the city's charter said, the lakefront "forever free, open and clear." For two decades he took on the unholy trinity of Chicago: greed, power and corruption, and despite constant vilification, he prevailed. What is now Grant Park got its name in 1901, and has been steadily improving ever since (with some time off in the 1970s when everything seemed to go to pot). Buckingham Fountain is one of the most magnificent in the world, and the nearby formal gardens are only getting better. At the south end, the Museum Campus has transformed what had been a car-clogged maze. Finally, despite contro-versy (see below), the urban wilderness of Northerly Island beckons those who want a respite from the crowded city.

● Start your walk at the southeast corner of E. Monroe St. and S. Columbus Dr. Diagonally cross the wide-open spaces of Butler Field, which is punctuated on the southwest corner by the Petrillo Bandshell. Before the launch of the stunning Pritzker Bandshell just north in Millennium Park, this was ground zero for events like the jazz and blues festivals. When Michael Jordan played for the Chicago Bulls and winning the NBA title was an annual affair, this was where hundreds of thousands would gather to celebrate the victory, even if they couldn't actually see anything due to the atrocious sightlines. The sound quality was equally bad; the entire area is better now that it has been relegated to second-string status.

● Take the landscaped course just east of the bandshell and cross E. Jackson Blvd. Deeply shaded and intricately laid out, this is the oldest and most formal area of Grant Park. From here south to Balbo Dr. the elegant Beaux Arts design beautifully recalls the idealism expressed by Daniel Burnham in his 1909 master plan for the city. The richness of the floral plantings has been much improved in recent years, and shows how far the Park District has come since the decades when workers thought "park" was something they should do with their butts.

● Rise up a few wide steps and you enter the pink-hued gravel expanse that surrounds one of the city's great icons: Buckingham Fountain. Donated to the city by Kay Sturges Buckingham in 1927 in memory of her brother, the thundering display of water draws crowds day and night during temperate months. The reflecting pool represents Lake Michigan and the four corner fountains the states on the lake. The 1.5 million gallons that go into the display spray in a planned progression that starts small. As each basin fills more jets are stimulated until the climax when the central fountain spurts up 150 feet. At night colored lights add to the show. Note that the fountain is due for some major work and may be closed. Fortunately Buckingham wisely left an endowment for this. Note also that fences have been erected to keep you from going directly across Lake Shore Dr. to the lake. This is a shame. Once there were stoplights here for the crosswalks, and many people felt the need to cool off after the stimulation of the fountain.

● Walk due west to the sidewalks along the eastern terminus of E. Congress Pkwy. and cross over the Metra train tracks. Prior to the triumph of the car, this was a pedestrian promenade that ended in grand steps down to Michigan Ave. Now you'll have to look past the idling buses to recall this more gracious period. Better yet, look up to the dual 17-foot-high statues of the *Bowman* and the *Spearman*. Cast in bronze in 1927 by Ivan Mestrovic, horse fetishists will appreciate the rather jaw-dropping anatomical correctness of the stallions.

● Follow the strip of the park south between S. Michigan Ave. and the walls shielding the train tracks. The Grant Park horticulturalists are in prime form here, with lavish and formal plantings that wouldn't look out of place at a French chateau. Just south of E. Harrison St., look for the *Spirit of Music*, a 1923 statue of a bare-breasted woman holding a lyre. It is backed by carved panels showing the Chicago

Symphony Orchestra. These panels went missing for several decades after some boneheaded park employee dumped them in the lake.

- At E. 9th St. climb the hill (directions uncommon in Chicago) to the monument of Gen. John Logan. This is a fine example of the kind of monumental civic expression that was common in Chicago's early days, and which has not withstood the test of time. The stallion the general straddles sets the standard for realistic depiction of horse anatomy found elsewhere in the park. Logan himself was less impressive. He was a moderately successful commander in the Civil War. Later, he was a Republican senator from Illinois for over 12 years. Logan was known for his violent rhetoric and brutal political assaults on opponents. He might have lived 100 years too soon.

- A new walkway goes due south from Logan and links up with another example of the good work being done in the park today: a new entrance from E. 11th St. that leads to a pedestrian bridge over the Metra tracks. As you walk take time to appreciate the careful layout and detailing that fully honor the park's classical roots. Once over the tracks, pause and look south to the Metra Roosevelt Rd. station. For decades this was a despicable dump that brought shame onto every public body responsible for it. By 2010 it should finally be replaced by something more in line with its grand surroundings.

- Continue east on the bridge and then take the curving walk that goes down and under S. Columbus Dr. On the other side, immediately walk south to the statue of the road's namesake, Christopher Columbus. Looking optimistically ahead ("That's India, I know it!"), Columbus wears heavy duds typical

Classic view from east of the Shedd Aquarium

of the era. Happily, the bronze doesn't capture the true essence of the man between his annual baths.

- From the Columbus statue, walk north over the grass to the wide walkway that leads to the museum campus. This entire area bears no resemblance to its appearance just a few years ago when the northbound lanes of Lake Shore Dr. ran between the Field Museum and the Shedd Aquarium, creating a traffic-choked island. When LSD was consolidated in the 1990s this entire portion of Grant Park was reconfigured with it. Undulating relief was brought to the previously flat parklands and thousands of trees were planted. It's a fine addition to Grant Park overall, although you might wish the Park District would plant a few more benches to go with the oaks.

- Promenade through the wide pedestrian Lake Shore Dr. underpass to the Museum Campus and take the south fork to the Field Museum. Take a break from the weather (sunny, hot, cold, snowy, etc.) in the grand central hall that bisects the building. Within this soaring public space even Sue, the 13-foot-high and 42-foot-long skeleton of a toothy Tyrannosaurus rex looks small—well, not that small.

- Exit back out the north entrance of the Field and cross the plaza to the Shedd Aquarium. Look for various fishy features on the exterior. Inside the exhibits are literally whale-sized; the beluga whales in the Oceanarium enjoy sweeping lake views and continue to breed, even as debate continues about the ethics of keeping them captive. Facing the main entrance, walk down and around to the left so you can follow the watery curves of the sweeping walkway east.

- Stroll the lakefront promenade straight east for 500 yards to the Adler Planetarium. There are no points awarded if you suddenly stop and say: "Gosh, I should take a photograph." The views north to the heart of the city are the dream of every lethargic postcard producer. At the Adler, look for the 12 signs of the zodiac on each of the 12 sides of the original granite building. Inside the entrance, an original panel records the eight known planets of our solar system at the time of the Adler's opening in 1930. For years, a little addendum had to explain the absence of the supposed ninth planet Pluto, which had yet to be discovered. Fortunately time heals all wounds, and with the demotion of Pluto to the status of non-planet the panel is accurate again.

- From the Adler, take the narrow walk down to the 12th St. Beach. Despite the popularity of the Museum Campus, this pristine crescent of sand still feels almost private most days. A spiffy new beach house adds class for those needing relief.

- At the south end of the beach, cut around behind the Charter One Pavilion, a temporary open-air performance venue with a name that's bound to change with the whims of corporate sponsorship. Walk a bit west over the grass and you'll find a path that runs south through the heart of Northerly Island. If you think that building off to the east looks like a pint-sized airport terminal you'd be right.

  From 1947 until 2003 the island was better known as Meigs Field, a pipsqueak of an airport much-loved by execs who could get from the seat of their company plane to the seat in their Loop office in a matter of minutes. In the 1990s Mayor Daley—normally a close chum of the corporate crowd—proposed converting the island into a park, a use that had been called for under Burnham's 1909 plan. Much wrangling followed, and Daley's plans were stymied until he literally bulldozed the opposition. Under cover of darkness city crews cut huge holes in the runway, effectively closing the airport and stranding more than a dozen planes. The outrage was predictable, and Daley offered a litany of justifications, including the now-stock excuse for government malfeasance: post-9/11 security concerns. The concrete soon disappeared, replaced by 91 acres of prairie flowers and grasses. Little more has been built as the island figures prominently in the city's bid for the 2016 Olympics and plans are fluid. In the meantime, Northerly Island is the largest place in the city for an idyllic escape. Few people come out here, and as you meander the 1½ miles of paths you are rewarded with views of the Loop across an ocean of purple and pink wildflowers.

- The 146 Outer Drive Express bus connects back through the Museum Campus to the Loop.

CONNECTING THE WALKS

To link up with Burnham Park and the lakefront south, walk west around Burnham Harbor to a point roughly opposite the old terminal and pick up Walk 5. Going north, Walk 16 starts across E. Monroe St. and follows the lakefront across the Chicago River.

POINTS OF INTEREST

Field Museum www.fieldmuseum.org, 1400 S. Lake Shore Dr., 312-922-9410

Shedd Aquarium www.sheddaquarium.org, 1200 S. Lake Shore Dr., 312-939-2426

Adler Planetarium www.adlerplanetarium.org, 1300 S. Lake Shore Dr., 312-922-7827

ROUTE SUMMARY

1. Start at the southeast corner of E. Monroe St. and S. Columbus Dr.
2. Diagonally cross Butler Field.
3. Cross E. Jackson Blvd. and walk south through the landscaped gardens to Buckingham Fountain.
4. Walk due west to the sidewalks along the eastern terminus of E. Congress Pkwy. and cross over the Metra train tracks.
5. Follow the strip of the park south between S. Michigan Ave. and the walls shielding the train tracks.
6. At E. 9th St. climb the hill to the monument of Gen. John Logan.
7. Take the new walkway due south from the monument.
8. Take the pathway from E. 11th St. that leads to a pedestrian bridge over the Metra tracks.
9. Continue east on the bridge and then take the curving walk that goes down and under S. Columbus Dr.
10. On the other side, immediately walk south to the Christopher Columbus statue.
11. From the Columbus statue, walk north over the grass to the wide walkway that leads to the museum campus.
12. Go through the wide pedestrian Lake Shore Dr. underpass to the Museum Campus and take the south (right) fork to the Field Museum.
13. Cross the plaza to the Shedd Aquarium.
14. Follow the lakefront promenade straight east for 500 yards to the Adler Planetarium.
15. From the Adler, take the narrow walk down to the 12th St. Beach.
16. At the south end of the beach, cut around behind the Charter One Pavilion.
17. Walk west over the grass to a path that runs south through the heart of Northerly Island.

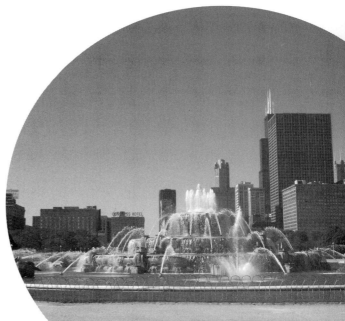

Buckingham Fountain

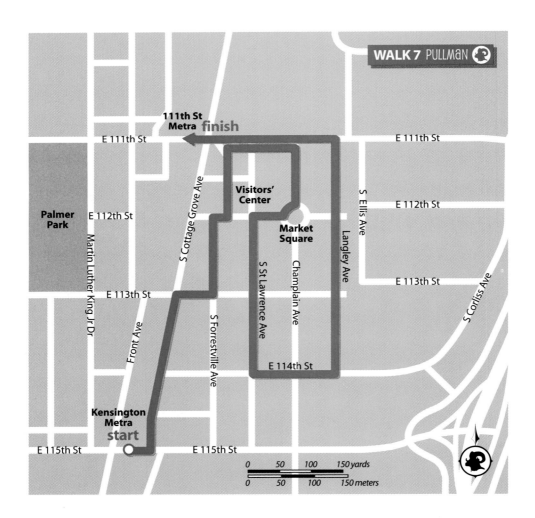

WALK 7 PULLMAN

111th St
Metra finish
E 111th St
E 111th St

Palmer Park
E 112th St
Visitors' Center
E 112th St

S Cottage Grove Ave
Market Square
S Ellis Ave

Martin Luther King Jr Dr
E 113th St
S St Lawrence Ave
Champlain Ave
Langley Ave
E 113th St

Front Ave
S Forrestville Ave
E 114th St
S Corliss Ave

Kensington Metra
start
E 115th St
E 115th St

0   50   100   150 yards
0   50   100   150 meters

7 PULLMAN: GO FOR a RIDE IN every CLASS

BOUNDARIES: **E. 11th St., S. Langley Ave., E. 115th St., S. Cottage Grove Ave.**
DISTANCE: **2.3 miles**
PUBLIC TRANSIT: **Metra Electric Blue Island Line and the South Shore Line trains to Kensington; 111 Pullman bus from the Red Line 95th El stop**

Pullman embodies the extremes of capitalism, good and bad. The neighborhood was built in the 1880s to house workers for George M. Pullman's Palace Car Company factory, which sprawled north of 111th St. On the surface it was a model community with a full range of amenities for residents, but its underpinnings were the same ferocious belief in profits that Pullman applied to all of his ventures. Every aspect of the admittedly beautiful town was meant to produce a return on investment, even the church. A recession led Pullman to cut his workers' wages in 1894, but there was no accompanying cut in the town's rents or the cost of food in the company stores. The workers called a strike, which ended in violent repression, and emotions remained raw for years after. When Pullman died in 1897 he was buried in an armored vault in Graceland Cemetery to prevent desecration of his corpse (see Walk 26). A year later the courts ordered the company to sell off the town. Meanwhile the politics of the area were radicalized and for many years residents regularly voted socialist.

The town's fortunes have followed the region's: an idiotic scheme in the 1960s to demolish Pullman for commercial use was only stopped at the last minute. The Pullman factory closed for good in 1981 and many other industries followed, causing great hardship. But through it all the inherent beauty of architect Solon S. Beman's designs have been undiminished. The neighborhood has an uncommon vibrancy for this part of the city. Many residents are lifers, and there's a remarkably diverse racial mix. As you walk the dozen blocks of Pullman you'll be struck both by its unique qualities that once inspired critics to call it the "world's most perfect town," and the unparalleled community pride.

● **Start the walk by ducking out of the Metra Kensington station and ducking under the tracks on E. 115th St. on the east side of the railway embankment. Note the Cal Harbor Restaurant one block farther on. It's a classic diner and your best bet for a meal in Pullman (the soup is tonic on a fall day). The name is drawn (!) from** the industrial body of water just east of here that has long been a drop-off spot for people who've run afoul of the Chicago mob.

- Turn north on S. Cottage Grove Ave., which runs from here almost 10 miles north nearly to downtown. While walking two blocks north, check out the row houses at 11307 S. Cottage Grove. Extra spiffy details such as round windows were meant to impress passengers—especially those in Pullmans—on passing trains. At the E. 113th St. underpass, behold the finely detailed indigo mural, the result of a community project to form bonds between Pullman and Roseland, the economically troubled community on the west side of the tracks.

- Walk one block east on E. 113th St. and turn north on S. Forestville Ave. The east side of the street presents the classic Pullman motif of finely detailed brick facades with just enough variation to maintain interest. Near the southwest corner with E. 112th St., a car wash occupies the tumbledown remains of the Pullman stables.

- Cross to the mundane 1950s cement-block low-rise, a former American Legion post that is now home to the Historic Pullman Visitor Center. Occasional guided tours leave from here, but you can pick up a self-guiding walking tour any time it's open (typically Tuesday to Sunday). Displays trace the history of both the town and the Pullman Company. One preserved ad from a company store proclaims "A Lot of Misses Rubbers, per pair 9¢." Note that this community-run visitor center is one of two often-competing organizations representing Pullman (see next bullet). For the best visit try to arrive when both are open.

- Plow across the grass—site of the old sky-lit shopping arcade—northeast to the town's jewel, the Hotel Florence. A Queen Anne pastiche, this 50-room hotel has an inviting wrap-around porch. Inside, it is slowly being restored back to its glory; you can see hints in the elaborate tiled flooring and ornate pressed tin ceiling. There's no food served, but the bar and its classic neon sign hold great promise for the future. This is the home of the other local organization, the Pullman State Historic Site, which manages the restoration of the hotel, surviving factory building, and the slow march to an eventual state-financed museum (the perilous finances of Illinois mean that won't be happening anytime soon). The historical displays in the hotel are

Back Story: a Company Life

In an interview with a Chicago newspaper in 1918, a Pullman worker described his life this way:

"We are born in a Pullman house, cradled in a Pullman crib, paid from a Pullman store, taught in a Pullman school, confirmed in a Pullman church, exploited in a Pullman shop. And when we die we'll be buried in a Pullman grave and go to Pullman hell."

excellent, and include recreated rooms. Note that normal hours are Monday to Friday, although you may be able to arrange visits on weekends.

● Cross E. 111th St.—the traditional boundary of residential Pullman—and enter (if you can) the Pullman factory site. From what remains it's difficult to grasp that this was once a sprawling complex of factories with a near monopoly on passenger car production during a time when railroads bought hundreds of cars annually. Known as the Clock Tower Building for obvious reasons, the administration building was gutted by fire in 1998 but recently rebuilt, although the state's money ran out before the planned museum could be built inside. If the gates are open, prowl around to get a feel for a fragment of a 19th-century factory. You might just emerge with an urge to unionize.

● From the factory site, walk south down S. Champlain Ave. to the plaza with E. 112th St. Four narrow buildings frame this beautiful square, which once had a market in the middle. The charred frame is all that's left of the second market to burn down here.

● Go one block west on 112th and stop in front of the Greenstone United Methodist Church, which is the oh-so-literal name for what was originally an all-faiths facility. The gorgeous exterior stones were imported from New England, and there's no proof that Pullman selected them because of the color of money. Inside there's some nicely carved trim, a large organ, and during the annual Fall home tours, you can get good homemade chili in the hall.

● Walk south on S. St. Lawrence Ave. Immediately across from the church is Dig It!, a store that's part garage sale and part hipster vintage boutique. Mid-block, the houses are a little more richly ornamented; these were where the skilled craftsmen lived. As you walk the streets you'll soon discern the company class system through the subtle variations in the houses. Skilled workers had fireplaces, laborers only stoves.

- As you cross E. 113th St., take in the somewhat shabby Pullman's Pub just in from the corner. But looks can be deceiving, and this neighborhood institution (a.k.a. Humberto's) serves up cold Old Style and recently cold (i.e., frozen) pizza to a jovial crowd of locals and regulars. Harrison Ford used the pay phone here while on the lam in 1993's *The Fugitive*. In 2001 numerous snowy scenes for the Tom Hanks and Paul Newman movie *The Road to Perdition* were filmed on the streets of Pullman.

- Go down one of the north-south running alleys to see the extraordinary variations of the homes behind the harmonious front façades. Decades of renovations and alterations on the rear of the houses present a rich tableau of stories. Keep your ears open for the cluck of the odd urban chicken.

- Turn east on E. 114th St. and go two blocks to S. Langley Ave. Turning north on the west side of the street you'll see some of the most unchanged original row houses in Pullman. You'd never suspect that 11322 had a stylish interior from its original and unadorned front. Look at the vintage details on the austere façades of 11314 and 11312. On the east side of the block, ponder the symmetry of the three-flat apartments which boasted private bathrooms.

- At the northeast corner with E. 112th St. there's one of two surviving "blockhouses," an apartment building for entry-level workers which featured but one bathroom per floor.

- There's a small park at the southeast corner of E. 111th St. Look for the interesting plaques with old aerial photos of the factories.

- Walk west on 111th. Notice how the homes on the south side are rather grand. These were for top managers, and their proximity to the factory meant that there would be no unnecessary mingling with the masses. The large house at 623 belonged to the company physician. A series of owners have spent the last three decades restoring it. Note that even the best houses in Pullman were semi-detached dwellings. For his part George Pullman lived in a mansion in the millionaire's neighborhood of Prairie Ave. south of the Loop (see Walk 13).

● **Continue west to the 111th St. Metra stop for trains back to the Loop. For South Shore trains you'll need to return to the Kensington Station.**

POINTS OF INTEREST

Cal Harbor Restaurant 546 E. 115th St., 773-264-5436

Historic Pullman Visitor Center www.pullmanil.org, 11141 S. Cottage Grove Ave., 773-785-8901

Hotel Florence/Pullman State Historic Site www.pullman-museum.org, 1111 S. Florence Ave., 773-660-2342

Dig It! 11208 S. St. Lawrence Ave., 773-520-1373

Pullman's Pub 611 E. 113th St., 773-568-0264

ROUTE SUMMARY

1. From the Kensington Metra station, cross under the tracks on E. 115th St. and turn left on S. Cottage Grove Ave.

2. Turn right and walk one block east on E. 113th St.

3. Turn left on S. Forestville Ave.

4. Cross the grass from the visitor center to the Hotel Florence.

5. Cross E. 111th St. and enter the Pullman factory site.

6. Exit the factory and walk south on S. Champlain Ave.

7. Turn right on E. 112th St.

8. Turn left on S. St. Lawrence Ave.

9. Turn left on E. 114th St. and go two blocks to S. Langley Ave.

10. Turn left and walk north to E. 111th St.

11. Turn left and walk west to the 111th St. Metra stop.

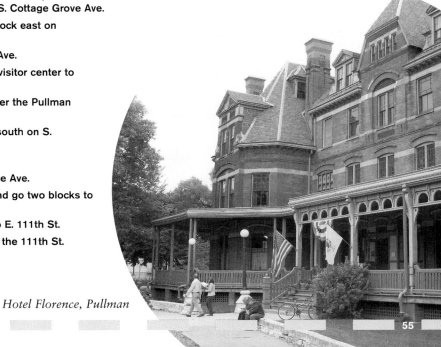

Hotel Florence, Pullman

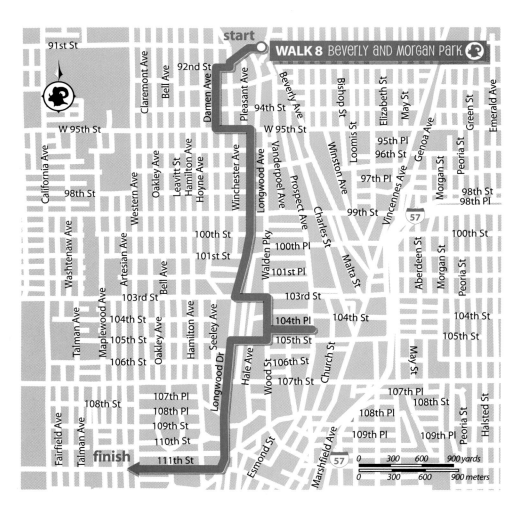

start

WALK 8 BEVERLY AND MORGAN PARK

finish

91st St
92nd St
94th St
W 95th St
95th Pl
96th St
97th Pl
98th St
98th Pl
99th St
100th St
100th Pl
101st Pl
103rd St
104th Pl
104th St
105th St
105th St
106th St
107th St
107th Pl
108th St
108th Pl
109th Pl
109th Pl

Claremont Ave
Bell Ave
Damen Ave
Pleasant Ave
Beverly Ave
Bishop St
Elizabeth St
May St
Green St
Emerald Ave
Peoria St
Genoa Ave
Morgan St

W 95th St
98th St

California Ave
Western Ave
Oakley Ave
Leavitt St
Hamilton Ave
Hoyne Ave
Winchester Ave
Longwood Ave
Vanderpoel Ave
Prospect Ave
Charles St
Winston Ave
Smith St
Loomis St
Vincennes Ave

100th St
101st St

Washtenaw Ave
Artesian Ave
Maplewood Ave
Bell Ave
Hamilton Ave
Seeley Ave
Walden Pky
Malta St
Aberdeen St
Morgan St
Peoria St

103rd St
104th St
105th St
106th St

Talman Ave
Oakley Ave
Longwood Dr
Hale Ave
Wood St
Church St
May St
Peoria St
Halsted St

107th Pl
108th Pl
109th St
110th St
111th St

Fairfield Ave
Talman Ave
Esmond St
Marshfield Ave

57

57

0   300   600   900 yards
0   300   600   900 meters

8 Beverly and Morgan Park: Head for the (Small) Hills

BOUNDARIES: **W. 91st Ave., S. Beverly Ave., W. 111th St., S. Western Ave.**
DISTANCE: **4 miles**
PUBLIC TRANSIT: **Metra Rock Island Line trains to 91st/Beverly and 111th**

Tens of thousands of years ago during an ice age, glaciers covered Chicago. One went a little wayward and ended up dumping its load of stone in a ridge under what are today the upscale communities of Beverly and Morgan Park. First developed in the 1870s and 1880s, some of the city's most eclectic mansions can be found here in what for Chicago qualifies as rolling terrain (okay, it's ripples in a bathtub, but still . . .). A stroll here is a suburban treat, and offers a good lesson in what can result when efforts are made to integrate neighborhoods. When block-busting (the act of real estate agents panicking white residents with racial fears, then buying their houses cheaply and reselling them for huge profits to African-Americans) became a problem in the 1950s and 1960s, community groups urged residents not to sell, while concurrently acting as boosters. It mostly worked, and today Beverly and Morgan Park are integrated to a degree found in few other parts of the city.

● Start your walk at the Beverly/91st St. Metra Station. Exit the parking lot to the right and turn west on W. 91st St. where you will get a preview of the architectural delights to come on your walk. The only house on the north side of the street is number 1826. Built in 1894, it's a gingerbread fantasy, and what with the Dan Ryan Woods stretching behind it, you might fully expect to hear the conniving growl of the Big Bad Wolf.

● Just west of 1826, 91st St. forks. Whether you take the high road or the low road, after 100 yards you'll end up on S. Winchester Ave. Go south slightly and head west on W. 92nd St. Strolling the blocks, you'll come to appreciate the symphony of architecture that gives Beverly and Morgan Park their charm. Tudor, Prairie, Craftsman, Queen Anne and French Provincial are just some of the styles that combine to form the genial pastiche.

- Turn south on S. Damen Ave., one of the city's major streets (it runs in fits and starts), named for Father Arnold Damen, an early Chicago priest thought to have a lot of clout with God as his prayers are credited with saving Holy Family Church (see Walk 12) from the Chicago fire. Stop in front of 9332. The triple gables make this one of the prettier Queen Annes on the street, but what makes it notable is that current Supreme Court Justice John Paul Stevens called this home for many years after World War II. Born in Chicago, Stevens's father built the world's largest hotel, the eponymous Stevens Hotel (now the Chicago Hilton and Towers) in the 1920s on S. Michigan Ave., only to be wiped out by the Depression. John Paul still managed to save money and get his law degree from Northwestern University, where he attained the highest GPA in the school's history. While living here he developed a sterling reputation for anti-trust litigation and his probity in investigating judicial corruption (which in Illinois is like mushroom-picking after a rain). He left Beverly in 1975 when Gerald Ford appointed him to the Supreme Court.

- At busy W. 95th St. (the main east-west artery for this part of the South Side) walk east on the north side of the street. Depending on your genetic proximity to a dog, your nose may lead you right to 1844, home of Jimmy Jamm Sweet Potato Pies. Just as you'd expect from the name, this is a cathedral of all things yam. Try a heavenly slice of pie for only $2.50. On summer and fall Sundays, there's a good farmers market in the parking lot on the southeast corner.

- Cross 95th (or play Russian roulette, which may be safer) and stroll south on S. Longwood Ave, which runs along the base of the ridge. This is the esthetic spine of the neighborhood. Some of the finest homes are found here amongst parks and the tree-shaded ridge, a ripple of gravel left over from glacial times. Because the ridge often had a bluish look in summertime haze, early settlers came to call it Blue Island for its appearance on the horizon. As developments started in the 1880s, the area gained the moniker "Beverly Hills," again because of the ridge. Given the Chicago landscape's close resemblance to a pancake, it's understandable that a geologic feature reaching up to 80 feet in height would be called a hill. As to the Beverly part, there's ongoing debate and no one is really sure. (At the time Beverly got its name, what's now Beverly Hills in California was still lima bean farms and didn't get its name until 1906.)

- Where W. 97th St. abuts Longwood, pause and ponder Ridge Park. Long popular with neighborhood kids, one old-timer gazed at it morosely and told us: "Before global warming ruined the weather, we used to flood it with water in the winter and ice-skate for months."

- At W. 99th St., check out the train station. It has recently undergone a restoration that takes it back to its original 1898 style, which might be described as "suburban precocious." All six Metra stations from 91st (where you arrived) to 111th form a historic district and honor the flair that the Rock Island Railroad gave their designs. Just south, look for Café Luna, which has good coffee, baked goods and a delightful back patio.

- Continue south on Longwood. The ridge becomes more pronounced south of W. 99th St. At 9914 look for the familiar bold horizontal lines of Frank Lloyd Wright. The house has held its regal position here since 1908, except for one major desecration: some owner—probably with rocks in their head—applied the fake stone façade you see over Wright's original stucco. This sort of fakery would have made Wright barf, although pretty much most aspects of ordinary life made him barf.

- On the southwest corner with W. 100th St., note Hurley Playlot Park. According to local lore, when plans leaked out that a Catholic Church was planned for this spot, the local WASP community hurriedly bought the plot and turned it into a park in order to keep to Catholics out of Beverly (welcome mats here before World War II were yanked almost as quickly for Irish-Catholics as they were for African-Americans). The

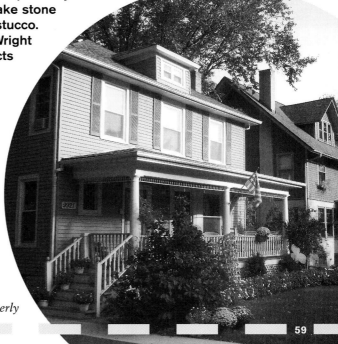

Typical comfy homes in Beverly

Catholics got their church anyway; St. Barnabas opened one block south in 1924 and Father Timothy Hurley was the first pastor. Later, as Irish-Americans came to dominate local affairs, they got pay-back by renaming the park for him.

● Stop at the intersection with W. 103rd St. If you hear the phrase "I fart in your general direction!" it may be coming from the fantasy castle to your immediate right. Built from local limestone as a family home in 1886, the crenellated turrets are right out of *Monty Python and the Holy Grail*. It's now a Unitarian church. East of Longwood, the Metra 103rd St. station anchors a darling little boutique and cafe-laden commercial strip. The World Music Company is a non-profit store that specializes in folk music as well as blues, jazz and more. You'll find gems here that have never been on iTunes as well as an enthusiastic staff. Watch for performances. Across the street, Hynes' Irish Cottage has all things old sod. Given that the recent performance of the locally beloved Fighting Irish football team at Notre Dame, it's fortunate that they stock a huge range of hankies.

● Walk east on W. 103rd St. to S. Wood St., turn south and then east on 104th Place (a.k.a. Walter Burley Griffin Place). One of Frank Lloyd Wright's most talented architects, Walter Burley Griffin started his own practice in 1906 and in 1911 married another Wright architect, Marion Lucy Mahony, one of America's first female architects, an early environmentalist and the regular winner of design competitions among Wright's staff. They proved to be quite a formidable design team; this block has several houses attributed to Griffin, including those at 1736, 1724, 1712 and 1666 (others were probably interpretations of his work by others). These innovative and compact houses sold for under $5,000, a bargain even in 1910.

● Return west via S. Wood St. and W. 105th St. Turn south and resume the long—albeit delightful—march down Longwood. Need a place for a wedding reception? The terraces at 10616 would do nicely—although a mis-thrown bouquet could be fatal. Behind the sturdy maroon walls, the Ridge Historical Society has changing exhibits that are open much less regularly than the placement of windows on the Longwood façade. The entrance faces S. Seeley Ave.

- W. 107th St. marks the northern border of Morgan Park proper.

- Addicts of cable shopping channels will thrill to the cute-as-a-button confection of a house at 10838. Architect Harry Hale Waterman designed the house for himself in 1892. The slightly exaggerated details evoke comparisons to portraits of doe-eyed puppies and the like. In fact, were Waterman alive today, he could probably make a fortune designing those treacley little collectible villages hawked around the clock on TV. His work can be found throughout the area, including around the corner at 2023 W. 108th Pl.

- Just before W. 111th St., at a spot no one finds funny, Bohn Park is a somber little plot of green. However, that's just as well, as it doesn't detract from the 111th St. Metra Station. With its Romanesque arch over the entrance, it's probably the most appealing of the Rock Island stations. It was lovingly restored in 2002 in time for the 150th anniversary of the first train that ran past here to Joliet.

- End your trip here and catch a train back to the Loop. Otherwise sample local culture high and low one-half mile west on S. Western Ave. Following 111th St. you'll see an especially banal collection of 1950s buildings, leaving you convinced that every architect with talent perished in the war. At the southwest corner of 111th and Western, the striking Beverly Arts Center has galleries, studios, and more. North and south of the intersection you'll find inspiration of a different sort: the "Stations of the Cross" are 12 bars on the west side of Western Ave. running from W. 99th St. to W. 119th St. (the east side is dry). All play heavily on faux Irish schtick; prime examples are the Dubliner and McNally's. For more South Side Irish culture, show up the Sunday before St. Patrick's Day for the legendary boozefest and raucous parade that runs from W. 103rd St. to W. 115th St.

POINTS OF INTEREST

Jimmy Jamm Sweet Potato Pies 1742 W. 99th St., 773-239-8990

Café Luna 1742 W. 99th St., 773-239-8990

World Music Company www.worldfolkmusiccompany.com, 1808 W. 103rd St.,
773-779-2546

Hynes' Irish Cottage 1907 W. 103rd St., 773-429-0666

Ridge Historical Society www.ridgehistoricalsociety.org, 10621 S. Seeley Ave.,
773-881-1675

Beverly Arts Center www.beverlyartcenter.org, 2407 W. 111th St., 773-445-3838

Dubliner 10910 S. Western Ave., 773-238-0784

McNally's 11136 S. Western Ave., 773-779-6202

route summary

1. Start at the Beverly/91st St. Metra Station.
2. Walk west on W. 91st St.
3. Turn left on S. Winchester Ave. and then turn right on W. 92nd St.
4. Turn left on S. Damen Ave.
5. Turn left on W. 95th St.
6. Turn right on S. Longwood Ave.
7. Turn left on W. 103rd St.
8. Turn right on S. Wood St. to 104th Place/Walter Burley Griffin Pl.
9. Retrace your steps on 104th Pl., jog south on S. Wood St. and turn right on W. 105th St.
10. Turn left on S. Longwood Ave.
11. End the walk at Bohn Park and the 111th St. Metra station, or optionally go west on W. 111th St. to S. Western Ave.

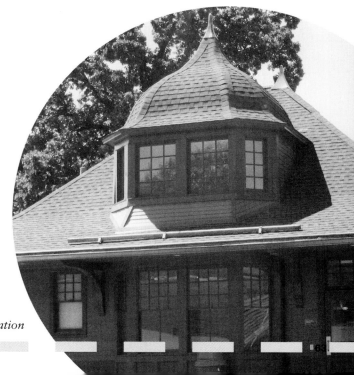

The recently restored 99th St. Metra Station

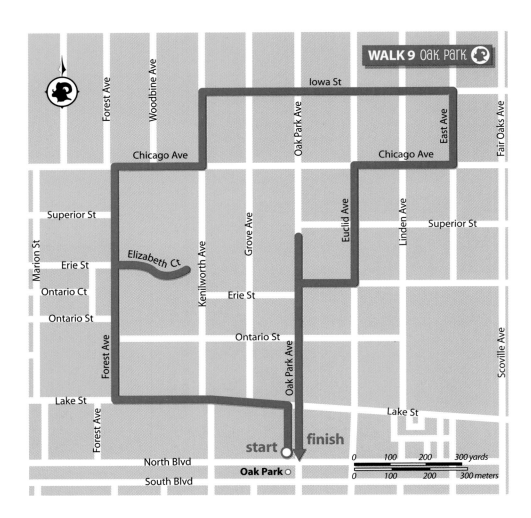

Forest Ave

Woodbine Ave

Iowa St

Oak Park Ave

East Ave

Fair Oaks Ave

Chicago Ave

Chicago Ave

Superior St

Euclid Ave

Linden Ave

Superior St

Marion St

Erie St

Elizabeth Ct

Kenilworth Ave

Grove Ave

Ontario Ct

Ontario St

Erie St

Forest Ave

Ontario St

Oak Park Ave

Scoville Ave

Lake St

Lake St

Forest Ave

start   finish

North Blvd

Oak Park

South Blvd

0   100   200   300 yards

0   100   200   300 meters

9 Oak Park: Wright and Wrong

BOUNDARIES: **Iowa St., East Ave., North Blvd., Forest Ave.**
DISTANCE: **2.7 miles**
PUBLIC TRANSIT: **Green Line El to Oak Park**

Although a pilgrimage for many spellbound by the legacy of Frank Lloyd Wright, Oak Park is also a delightful place to go for a stroll. The myriad architecturally significant buildings are but a bonus, and after a few blocks you'll begin to question the veracity of the oft-repeated quote attributed to local son Ernest Hemingway, who said Oak Park had "broad lawns and narrow minds." Let's face it, he was probably drunk. As for Wright, yes, he was America's greatest architect, and yes, he was an uncommon and original genius, but that's no reason for the hagiolatry on display by the vast crowd of architectural tourists, equipped with guidebooks and grim expressions, that throngs Oak Park's streets. Instead, have fun with Wright and Oak Park, enjoy his often-beautiful legacy while recalling that he was one of America's great characters.

● From the CTA Green Line El stop Oak Park, walk north one block on Oak Park Ave. This little commercial oasis features a number of good places for a meal, a drink, or a treat. Try the Pasta Shoppe and Cafe, a family-run restaurant that has good casual fare, a great patio and an extra "pe"—this being Oakke Parkke and all. On the west side of the street, Scoville Square has Prairie-style highlights. Within this handsome commercial block, consider a stop at the Magic Tree Bookshop. If you're traveling single you can pick up a puppet for company.

● Cross to the north side of Lake St. On the southwest corner of the intersection, look for the 1909 Horse Show Association Fountain. Much more modestly endowed than the stallions rearing up in Grant Park (see Walk 6), the horses here are part of a tableaux that celebrates the relationship of man and beast. Note the swell within the fountain sporting a tennis racket.

● Walk west along Scoville Park. A 1927 plaque notes that Oak Park's first "white" settler lived here on land purchased from the U.S. government for $1.25 an acre. Sort of like a mining entrepreneur today buying public lands for peanuts. Across the plaza, Oak Park's library (2003) offers plenty of ways to learn more about its famous residents. Note that the blocks immediately north of Lake St. are littered with many large apartment complexes from the aesthetically famished 1950s and 1960s. Should you stray from the route, watch where you look, or you might have a reaction much the same as Frank Lloyd Wright's.

- Continuing west, cross to the southeast corner of Lake and Kenilworth Ave., where lightning struck twice: first in 1905 when it caused a wooden church here to burn to the ground, and then metaphorically when Wright had his vision for a replacement. The resulting Unity Temple (1908) presents an image of an aloof and forbidding God to the street. Your passage inside is not made easy, and low ceilings inspire foreboding. But enter the temple and your spirits literally soar in a triumphant space brightly lit from the heavens via amber skylights above. It's widely regarded as one of Wright's true examples of genius.

- Back on Lake St., turn north on Forest Ave. Immediately on the right is the Oak Park Visitors Center, where you can get maps, audio guides, buy tickets for attractions and join a guided tour. It also sells lots of souvenir items Wright probably would have called "crap."

- Go north on Forest Ave. past the beautifully landscaped Austin Gardens, which must have received delivery of all those comfy benches missing from Chicago's parks. At the southwest corner with Ontario St. is a "memorial" to Wright by Egon Weiner that will surely make anyone who ever wanted to see his head on a stick exclaim: "Hot dog!"

- The next section of Forest Ave. to Chicago Ave. is thick with Wright treasures. Stern-faced acolytes abound. Going north, highlights follow by house number. Buildings not directly attributable to Wright are not credited to him. Contrast the gingerbready geegaws on 203 (1885) with the classic, Prairie-style understatement on the Wright-designed 210 (1901). Can these two be only 16 years apart? Five years later, Wright created the ochre-accented Beachy House at 238. He'd been hired to do a simple remodel on a cottage here, but got carried away. There's no record of what the owners did when they saw the bill.

- Turn east on Elizabeth Court. In 1909 Wright expressed his boldest design for the neighborhood yet with the assertive porches at number 6.

- Returning to Forest Ave., pause at the oddly stilted and turreted 1893 house at 300. The owner, Charles Purcell, who was no doubt peering across his wide lawn, is reported to have lamented that someone had better stop Wright before he ruined the entire street.

- It's worth taking a long pause in front of the wonder that is Wright's 1902 triumph at 318. He was always lauded for his attention to detail—note the exquisite horizontal banding on the walls and façade. The arched entrance is the perfect counterpoint, while the sedate roof provides a soft-spoken frame.

- Directly across from the serenity of 318, the Moore House on the southwest corner with Superior St. is a nightmare. Was FLW on LSD? Look for the plaque farther down Forest Ave. that shows the house as he designed it in 1895. Twenty-eight years later he was brought in for a remodel, and what you see is the result. Among the disturbing details are the strange gunport-like holes across the rear façade.

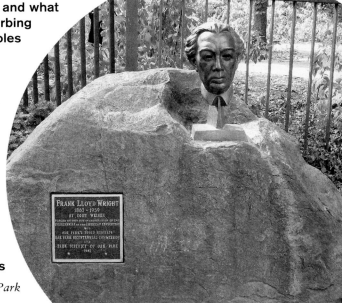

- Turn west on Chicago Ave. and go a few doors down to 1019. This simple Queen Anne was an early (1892) work Wright knocked off while moonlighting from his day job with the all-star firm of Adler and Sullivan. Although meant to be a simple cottage, his future philosophy was already apparent. For one, there were no closets, as he felt they ruined the purity of the interior space. Years later an owner had a disastrous sewage back-up, and it was

The head of Frank Lloyd Wright, Oak Park

BaCK STORY: He Was NOT a NICe MaN

Words like gracious, charming and generous are seldom found in descriptions of Frank Lloyd Wright unless they are preceded by a negative modifier. Typical is the story we were once told by a man pensively gazing at the Moore House. "I was 19 and going to a small architecture school back east. Wright came and spoke. Afterwards I tried to speak to him, because I admired him. He looked at me and said, 'You'll never be an architect, because you go to school in a shoe factory.' Then he hit me with his cane and drove away."

Typical of his arrogant outlook was Wright's response after he dumped his first wife and six kids to abscond to Europe in 1908 with a client's wife, Mamah Borthwick Cheney. Not waiting for a divorce, he left Oak Park for good and set up house (and studio) with Cheney in Wisconsin. In 1911 he tried to damp down public condemnation by holding a press conference on Christmas Day in which he proclaimed that as a "thinking man" he wasn't bound by the moral strictures of "ordinary men." Condemnation continued.

In 1914 Cheney, her two children, and four workers were bludgeoned by a deranged servant. Subsequently Wright took up with Miriam Noel, a morphine addict who'd sent him a sympathy card. In 1922 he finally pried a divorce out of his first wife and married Noel in 1923. In 1925 he showed his proclivity for more personal multi-tasking by having a child with Olga Ivanovna. He divorced Noel in 1927 and married Olga in 1928.

Were he alive today, Wright's tart tongue might well have allowed him a career as a yakker on cable television or talk radio. At his acerbic best he could succinctly summarize a situation, as when he was on a tour of the University of Notre Dame and was asked his opinion of the school's pride and joy, a new academic building. His response: "Plant ivy and hope it grows." But more often he was simply petty and mean. After two of his protégées, Walter Burley Griffin and Marion Mahony Griffin, married and achieved their own professional fame (see Walk 8), a jealous Wright would only refer to these acclaimed architects as "draughtsmen."

discovered that the sewer had never been properly implemented. Wright may have been an perfectionist with the small details but he was always known for having little interest in the mundane.

- Return east to the Frank Lloyd Wright Home and Studio at the southwest corner of Forest and Chicago avenues. It's well worth the time for the guided tour of the place where Wright lived and worked until he skipped town for good. Outside, the studio bears an odd resemblance to a D-Day pillbox; inside it is much more masterful in execution. Also note that Wright—who loved to prattle on about respecting the purity of materials—did things here like paint pipe so that it looked like mahogany.

- Walk one block east on Chicago Ave. to Kenilworth Ave., and on the north side of the street cross the plaza between the elaborate playground and Holmes School to the stub-end of Kenilworth. Go one block to the northeast corner with Iowa St. The house here indeed does have a moderately wide lawn. It's the boyhood home of Ernest Hemingway, who lived here from ages 6 to 18. Today it's refreshingly ordinary: a window air-conditioner drones on in summer, a Weber grill awaits weenies.

- You've now got a pleasant five-block stroll west on Iowa through the "real" (as in non-postcard-appearing) Oak Park. Turn south on East Ave. and go to the northwest corner with Chicago Ave. In 1950 this mannered, L-shaped house was purchased by Percy Julian, a brilliant chemist from Chicago who couldn't seem to ever find a job for one reason: he was black. He finally got a job as research director with the Glidden Company in Chicago. It was a time when even one black family moving into a Chicago neighborhood was enough to spark riots. Oak Park thought it was different, but on Thanksgiving Day 1950, gas was poured on the Julian home when no one was there. (That was the Oak Park difference: in Chicago they killed you in your living room; here they simply burned down your living room.) A year later the front lawn was dynamited, and Julian—one of the 20th century's most brilliant chemists—took to sitting in his tree out front with a shotgun. To many locals' credit, however, a group of more than 200 formed to support the Julians, and regularly stood out front chanting "welcome!" The family ended up living here for many years.

- Go two blocks west on Chicago Ave. and turn south on Euclid Ave. The next few blocks sport some truly vast mansions by a variety of architects. Most date from roughly 1880 to 1910. At 321, try to peek through the windows to see a young Wright's 1896 interior remodel of this grand 1883 home. If nothing else, the leaded windows are a hint at things to come. You'll have to peer around the back of the property at 317 to see Wright's one and only stable. Another early commission (1896), it is proof that everyone starts small. A 1929 conversion turned what must have been a very dark barn into a very dark house.

- Turn west on Erie St. and walk one block to Oak Park Ave. Go less than a block north to number 339, an extravagant Queen Anne vision in wood that was the birthplace of Ernest Hemingway in 1899. Displays inside document the cast of characters that made up his family.

- Return south two blocks to the Ernest Hemingway Museum at the northeast corner with Ontario St. This stolid hulk is stuffed with Hemingway ephemera. Nearby outdoor cafes feed off his legacy; for some reason none are named "Death in the Afternoon."

- Continue south and you can return to the CTA Green Line El stop.

POINTS OF INTEREST

Pasta Shoppe and Cafe 116 N. Oak Park Ave., 708-763-0600

Magic Tree Bookstore 141 N. Oak Park Ave., 708-848-0770

Oak Park Library 834 Lake St., 708-383-8200

Unity Temple 875 Lake St., 708-383-8873

Oak Park Visitors Center 158 Forest Ave., 708-848-1500

Frank Lloyd Wright Home and Studio www.wrightplus.org, 951 Chicago Ave., 708-848-1976

Ernest Hemingway Birthplace and Museum www.ehfop.org, 339 Oak Park Ave. and 200 Oak Park Ave., 708-524-5383

rouTE SummarY

1. From the CTA Green Line El stop Oak Park, walk north one block on Oak Park Ave.

2. Cross to the north side of Lake St.

3. Turn left and walk west along Scoville Park.

4. Cross to the southeast corner of Lake and Kenilworth Ave.

5. Continue west on Lake St.

6. Turn right on Forest Ave. and walk north.

7. Turn right on Elizabeth Court.

6. Return to Forest Ave. turn right, and head north.

7. Turn left on Chicago Ave. and walk to number 1019.

8. Head back east on Chicago to Kenilworth Ave. On the north side of the street cross the plaza between the elaborate playground and Holmes School to the stub-end of Kenilworth. Go one block to the northeast corner with Iowa St.

9. Turn right on Iowa St. and walk five blocks east.

10. Turn right on East Ave. and go one block.

11. Turn right on Chicago Ave. and walk two blocks west.

12. Turn left on Euclid Ave.

13. Turn right on Erie St. and walk one block to Oak Park Ave.

14. Turn right; go less than a block north to number 339.

15. Return south on Oak Park Blvd. to the CTA Green Line El stop.

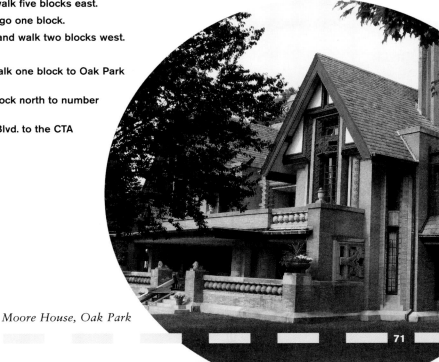

Moore House, Oak Park

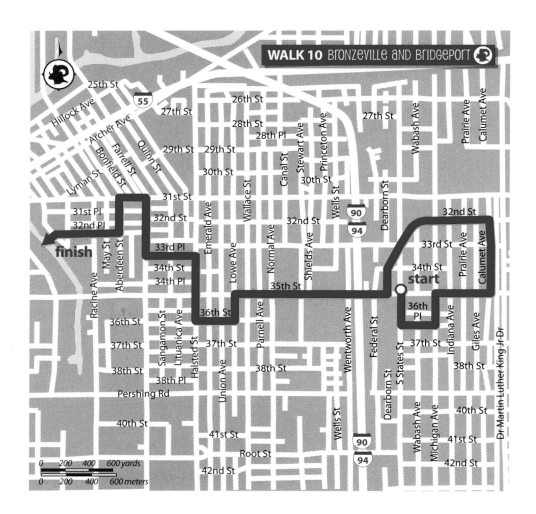

25th St

Hillock Ave

Archer Ave

Farrell St

Bonfield St

Lyman St

Quinn St

31st Pl

32nd Pl

finish

May St

Aberdeen St

Racine Ave

26th St

27th St

28th St

28th Pl

29th St   29th St

30th St

31st St

32nd St

33rd Pl

34th St

34th Pl

Emerald Ave

Wallace Ave

Canal St

Stewart Ave

Princeton Ave

30th St

32nd St

Normal Ave

Lowe Ave

Shields Ave

35th St

36th St

Wells St

27th St

Wabash Ave

Prairie Ave

Calumet Ave

90
94

Dearborn St

32nd St

33rd St

34th St

start

36th Pl

Prairie Ave

Calumet Ave

Indiana Ave

Giles Ave

Dr Martin Luther King Jr Dr

36th St

37th St

38th St

Sangamon St

Lituanica Ave

Halsted St

38th Pl

Pershing Rd

40th St

37th St

Union Ave

38th St

Parnell Ave

41st St

Root St

42nd St

Wells St

Wentworth Ave

Federal St

Dearborn St

S States St

37th St

38th St

90
94

Wabash Ave

Michigan Ave

40th St

41st St

42nd St

0   200   400   600 yards

0   200   400   600 meters

55

10 Bronzeville and Bridgeport: NOT TWO B'S IN a POD

BOUNDARIES: **31st St., S. Calumet Ave., 36th Place, Bubbly Creek**
DISTANCE: **4½ miles**
PUBLIC TRANSIT: **Green Line El to 35th-Bronzeville-IIT**

For decades residents of Bronzeville and Bridgeport avoided each other's neighborhoods. Although right next to each other, the first was black and the second white; the worst violence in the 1919 race riots centered on these two. Bronzeville was the heart of African-American culture in Chicago. But after World War II, it was also home to horrific public housing projects, and was in deep decline. In contrast, Bridgeport was the heart of Chicago's white power structure. After Mayor Richard J. Daley died in 1976, however, it too went into decline. But now gentrification, as well as Hispanic immigrants and the influence of Chinatown from the northeast, has given it new vitality, even as the faces in windows are less monochromatic. Bronzeville is also enjoying a resurgence thanks to investment and rising property prices. This walk combines interesting parts of both, a sacrilegious thought just a few years ago.

● **Exit the Green Line El at the 35th/Bronzeville stop. Look to your right as you face 35th St. and you'll see a Starbuck's at the intersection. There could be no more stark example of how this area has changed. This was the northern edge of the notorious Stateway Gardens public housing complex that ran south to Pershing Road where it abutted the even more notorious Robert Taylor Homes, which stretched to 54th St. All together there were 34 16- and 17-story concrete high-rises forming a single-file row down the east side of the Dan Ryan Expressway. Called a gulag for the poor by some and worse by others, the projects were home to the worst evils of society, as well as a myriad personal triumphs. The residents have been scattered and the projects replaced by mixed-income housing.**

● **Walk south on S. State St. At 3617 look for the name "Overton Hygienic Company" over the door. This was the headquarters of Anthony Overton, an African-American entrepreneur before World War II. The impressive terra-cotta tile outside has been restored for the building's use as business incubator. Just south at 3647 is the**

Chicago Bee Branch library. Overton published the *Chicago Bee*, a newspaper serving the black population. He's credited with promoting the term Bronzeville to describe the South Side at the suggestion of his drama critic. It was seen as a more flattering moniker than "black ghetto," which was used by the *Tribune* and other papers.

- Dart east on 36th Pl. and turn north on S. Michigan Ave. On your left is modern HQ for the Chicago Police. Go inside and jump through a few hoops to see the Haymarket Statue (see Walk 11). Turn east on E. 35th St. This formerly derelict part of town has found some of its old vitality, and the commercial strip is on the upswing. If the scores of teenagers you see scurrying about look a little serious, it's because two of the academically toughest high schools in Chicago are here. De LaSalle Institute, a Catholic boys school (the girls are safely stashed on the other side of the Dan Ryan), is on S. Michigan north of E. 35th St; the Chicago Military Academy is a co-ed public school with suitably tough standards housed partly in the old 1915 National Guard armory on S. Giles Ave. south of E. 35th St.

- Turn north on S. Calumet Ave. Although much has been lost, this part of Chicago once had a plethora of stone buildings rich in Romanesque details. Today the street has some gems amidst the holes; among the notable survivors are those at 3356-3360, 3322 and 3314-3316. You won't be able to help stopping to take in the row houses from 1894 at 3213-3219. The dramatic rooflines and intricate detailing are sure signs that this is the work of Frank Lloyd Wright.

- Head west on E. 32nd St. Pause as you cross S. Indiana Ave. and look one block south. If you're lucky, your heart won't break. The charred shell you see is all that remains after a tragic 2006 fire at the Pilgrim Baptist Church, the beautiful former synagogue that was the birthplace of gospel music in the 1930s. Mahalia Jackson and Aretha Franklin are just two of the singers who performed here. Steel shores up the walls while a decision is made on rebuilding.

- Try to imagine yourself as an embryo in an egg as you cross S. Michigan Ave. and enter the campus of the Illinois Institute of Technology, an incubator of numerous theories including Modernism, the classic steel and glass form found throughout the world and expressed at its highest in the Sears Tower. Formed from several cut-rate engineering schools after World War II, IIT gained the genius of Mies van der Rohe and his Bauhaus disciples when he was named head of the school's architecture department. He was put in charge of planning a new campus, and what resulted is a gem. As you wander the sidewalks, you'll see forms that gained universal acceptance. Maybe, in this nurturing environment, you'll hatch something yourself.

- Follow E. 32nd St until you near the El tracks and cut through the angular modern building that sits under the tracks and a huge circular acoustic baffle. The McCormick Tribune Campus Center (no, it wasn't donated by the *Sun-Times*) opened in 2003 and is the center of life for a campus that often lacked same. At any time a good number of the 4,500 undergrads and grad students are here cramming, laughing, eating or lost in iTunes. You can get a good free campus map here.

- Exit onto 33rd St. and cross S. State St. Walk diagonally southwest across the grassy commons and turn toward the low building of charcoal metal and glass directly south. S. R. Crown Hall (1956) is one of the most honored buildings in the United States. Fittingly, it is home to the College of Architecture. It seems so simple, but the longer you look at it the more you see. One vast open space inside, notice how the proportions all relate to each other just so while the entire structure seems to float over its translucent glass base.

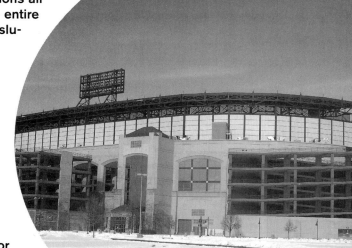

- Just west of Crown, follow the wide sidewalk due south to W. 35th St. Turn right and cross the Dan Ryan Expressway. Try not to sneer too much at the looming U.S. Cellular Field, the replacement for the much-loved and much-missed Comisky Park. The original ballpark stood south of the modern behemoth in what is now a vast wasteland of parking. In fact the entire area is a vast wasteland. When the rest of major

Ugly Comisky Park (U.S. Cellular Field)

league baseball was moving to quirky, fan-friendly stadiums integrated into the urban fabric (hop the Red Line up to Wrigley Field to see the original), Jerry Reinsdorf—owner of the White Sox—was building *this*. Cut around the elevator box/ticket windows to "Gate 5" to see the sad memorial to the home plate of the old Comisky. Gone is the gritty charm that made the Sox the favorite of so many, the under-dog vibe that came through in the fan's propensity to brawl, the goofy ownership of Bill Veeck, the propensity of Babe Ruth to nip across the street for a toot between double-headers. It's all gone, even the mangy watering holes, replaced by an ocean of asphalt. Can you really imagine fans spontaneously gathering here to celebrate a Sox victory away? They'd be mowed down by a speeding sand truck on 35th.

- Don't expect your spirits to lift heading west. The very long W. 35th St. viaduct under a slew of major train lines is dark, noisy, and often noxious. Fortunately, there is light at the end of the tunnel.

- Stop at the southeast corner of 35th and S. Lowe Ave. It should be no surprise that the city built both a small police station and a firehouse here when you realize who lived just down the block. Meantime, note that the cop shop was used extensively during the filming of the under-rated Jimmy Stewart 1948 docu-drama *Call Northside 777*. And check out the sweet little planter with kids' figurines in front of the firehouse.

- Walk south on S. Lowe Ave. to 3536. This was the longtime home of Mayor Richard J. Daley, the boss of all political bosses. A lifelong Bridgeport resident (he was born steps away at 3602 S. Lowe and died at his city hall desk in 1976), Daley was a state senator and a rising cog in the Chicago machine when he and his wife "Sis" had this bungalow built in 1939. They raised seven kids here, including the current mayor and William, a former U.S. secretary of commerce. Until the death of Sis in 2003, there was always a police car parked out front, lest any patronage seeker cause a ruckus. If the bungalow at first seems especially humble, note the details and finishes that set it apart from its truly humble neighbors.

- Continue south on Lowe and turn west on W. 36th St. Where the barking of dogs or the sizzle of steaks might be the aural hallmarks of some neighborhoods, in

Bridgeport you'll hear folks sitting out on their stoops, sharing the latest gossip with neighbors while accentuating their "dees" and "dohs" in the local dialect.

- Turn north on S. Halsted St, the not-so-thriving commercial center of the 'hood. Ramova's Grill is a timeless, Formica-countered dive with killer homemade chili. This is a fine place to order up a mother-in-law, one of the stalwarts of Chicago's stable of improbable junk foods. (A mother-in-law is so named because like the real kind they are likely to cause heartburn. Variations abound, but typically there's a corn tamale topped with chili and any of the myriad Chicago hot-dog fixings. Some places serve the oozing bomb in a hot-dog bun but not Ramova's.)

- After pausing to burp, continue north on S. Halsted St. For a congenial draft with old-timers, stop off at Mitchell's. Turn west on W. 33rd Pl. Amidst the timeless blue-collar bungalows and two-flats, a spate of recent fill-ins stand out like fake Rolexes. Expect to pay $700,000 or more for a 2.5-story, four-bedroom Bridgeport McMansion.

- Walk north on S. Morgan Ave. to busy W. 31st St. Take caffeine-sustenance at the Bridgeport Coffee House, the watering hole for a new generation of locals.

- Go west on 31st. There's no better sign of the neighborhood changes than at 1035, where the former Presbyterian church is now the Ling Shen Ching Tze Temple. Just next door, Immaculate Conception Church was built in 1909 by a German congregation.

- Turn south on S. Aberdeen St. and stop at W. 32nd St. On the corner, the classic façade of Pomierski Funeral Home fronts the final resting spot for generations of locals. Note the admonishment: "Flowers in Rear." In the middle of the block, St. Mary of Perpetual Help Church has Polish inscriptions that reveal the ethnicity of its original parishioners. Chicago easily supported dozens of huge churches like big-domed St. Mary's and Immaculate Conception in such close proximity because—brotherly love aside—you would *never* be caught dead in another ethnic group's church.

- Dart one block south and then head west on W. 32nd Place. For the first three blocks, the houses are the usual unassuming Bridgeport mix. But as you cross S. Throop St., suddenly things get upscale in a literally big way. This is the northern edge of the now-notorious Bridgeport Village development that built 110 flashy homes on former industrial land starting in 2004. Now the subject of FBI investigations, allegations about the development include payoffs, kick-backs, threats, and collusion by insiders at City Hall. The project itself is bankrupt and it's clear that something is amiss as the new developer-built streets are already crumbling. When you reach the river, be sure not to fall in. This is the notorious Bubbly Creek made famous by Upton Sinclair in *The Jungle* as one of the most befouled waterways in America. Although the packing houses that dumped decades of waste into it are long gone, bubbles still swirl up from the nastiness below. Some things in Chicago never change.

- Walk back three-quarters of a mile to Halsted to catch a No. 8 bus north to the Orange Line Halsted El stop or beyond or walk east and then south on S. Racine Ave. to catch a No. 35 35th St. bus back to Bronzeville.

POINTS OF INTEREST

Illinois Institute of Technology www.iit.edu, 3300 S. Federal St., 312-567-3000

Chicago White Sox chicago.whitesox.mlb.com, 333 W. 35th St., 312-674-1000

Ramova's Grill 3510 S. Halsted St., 773-847-9058

Mitchell's 3356 S. Halsted St., 773-927-6073

Bridgeport Coffee Company 3101 S. Morgan St., 773-247-9950

ROUTE SUMMARY

1. Exit the Green Line El at the 35th/Bronzeville stop.
2. Walk south on S. State St.
3. Turn left on 36th Place.
4. Turn left on S. Michigan Ave.
5. Turn right on 35th St.
6. Turn left on S. Calumet Ave.
7. Turn left on E. 32nd St.
8. Follow E. 32nd St. until you near the El tracks, and cut through the McCormick Tribune Campus Center.

9.   Exit onto 33rd St. and cross S. State St.

10. Walk diagonally southwest across the grassy commons to S. R. Crown Hall.

11. Just west of Crown, follow the wide sidewalk due south to W. 35th St.

12. Turn right and cross the Dan Ryan Expressway and continue through the long railroad viaduct.

13. Turn left on S. Lowe Ave.

14. Turn right on W. 36th St.

15. Turn right on S. Halsted St.

16. Turn left on W. 33rd Place.

17. Turn right on S. Morgan Ave.

18. Turn left on W. 31st.

19. Turn left on S. Aberdeen St.

20. Head right on W. 32nd Place until you reach the creek.

21. Walk back three-quarters of a mile to Halsted to catch a No. 8 bus north to the Orange Line Halsted El stop or walk east, then south on S. Racine Ave. to catch a No. 35 35th St. bus back to Bronzeville.

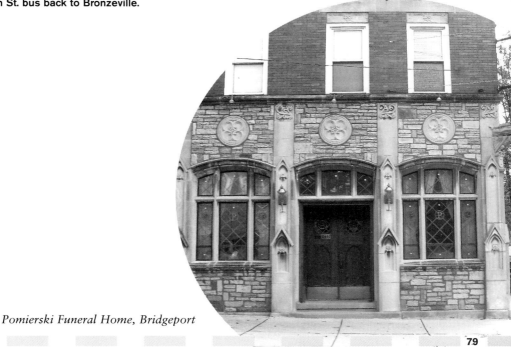

Pomierski Funeral Home, Bridgeport

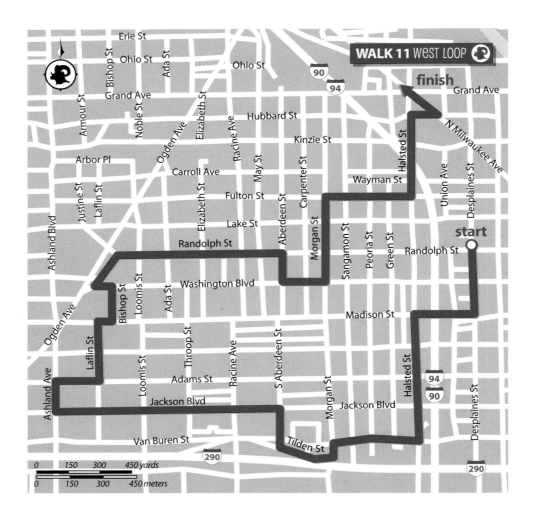

finish

start

Erie St
Bishop St
Ohio St
Ada St
Ohio St
Grand Ave
Hubbard St
Grand Ave
Arbor Pl
Carroll Ave
Kinzie St
N Milwaukee Ave
Armour St
Noble St
Elizabeth St
Racine Ave
May St
Carpenter St
Wayman St
Halsted St
Union Ave
Desplaines St
Ogden Ave
Justine St
Laflin St
Elizabeth St
Fulton St
Lake St
Randolph St
Sangamon St
Peoria St
Green St
Randolph St
Ashland Blvd
Washington Blvd
Aberdeen St
Morgan St
Ogden Ave
Bishop St
Loomis St
Ada St
Madison St
Laflin St
Throop St
Racine Ave
S Aberdeen St
Halsted St
Ashland Ave
Loomis St
Adams St
Morgan St
Jackson Blvd
Jackson Blvd
Van Buren St
Tilden St
90
94
94
90
290
290

0   150   300   450 yards
0   150   300   450 meters

11 WeST LOOP: MaYDaY ON MaY DaY

BOUNDARIES: **W. Grand Ave., Des Plaines St., Eisenhower Expressway, Ashland Ave.**
DISTANCE: **4.1 miles**
PUBLIC TRANSIT: **Green and Pink Lines El to Clinton**

In the sunrise shadow of the Loop, the West Loop has always been its Rodney Dangerfield uncle. And indeed it does get no respect; few know that events here in 1886 were the start of May Day commemorations the world over. Its many workaday neighborhoods have been home to scores of immigrants, notably Greeks. Its industrial blocks have supplied Chicago's best restaurants for generations, and amidst the rabble you can still find some stunning 1880s homes as well as the professional home of the richest woman in America.

Home to numerous trendy boutiques and upscale shops, this buyer's boulevard is well stocked with art, fashion and food. Just be sure to bring all your spare change—and maybe a piece of plastic or two.

● **Start your walk at the otherwise mundane intersection of W. Randolph St. and N. Des Plaines Ave. Amidst the spasmodic development look for the monument near the northeast corner. Dedicated in 2004, it is a representation of a speaker's wagon by Mary Brogger and recalls the events on this site in 1886. May 1 that year was the date unions had set for the imposition of an eight-hour work day. Rallies were held across North America, but the largest were in Chicago. Things were tense and skirmishes broke out at some factories when police opened fire on laborers. On the night of May 4, a large rally took place at this corner, which was then a busy area called Haymarket. A succession of speakers were interrupted when someone threw a bomb, killing a cop instantly. Scores more on both sides died in the violence that followed. Later, eight men were accused of the bombing, and four were hanged after highly dubious trials. A memorial to the police placed on the site had a checkered life (see sidebar). Development and the Kennedy Expressway erased any trace of the Haymarket. A planned "labor park" for the site has so far only yielded the Brogger sculpture. Few of those working long hours in the surrounding buildings have any idea that not only is this corner significant in the development of the eight-hour work**

Back Story: Statue Anarchy

In 1889, the city erected a statue to commemorate the cops killed in the Haymarket riot. Compared to the current statue on the site, it was decidedly single-minded in its representation: a lone policeman standing with arm upraised while demanding "peace in the name of the people of Illinois." Although few ever got this message as the plaques were stolen frequently. And it's doubtful whether they would have made a difference anyway to scores of people through the years who saw the "peace" command as a taunt. In the early 1900s a bus driver suddenly veered off his route and rammed the statue. He later said he was sick of seeing it every day. Re-erected, the statue was regularly the focus of protest marches, so in 1928 the city moved it—and it was hoped the

headaches—to Union Park several blocks west at N. Ashland Ave. But it remained the focus of more than pigeons, especially in 1969 and 1970 when it was twice blown up by radicals. Repaired yet again, the statue was first moved to the old Chicago Police headquarters on S. State St. and then to the courtyard of the Chicago Police Training Center on W. Jackson St. in 1976. This finally brought the statue a modicum of peace, yet its wanderlust days were not over. When the new police headquarters opened in Bronzeville at 3510 S. Michigan Ave. (see Walk 10) in 2000, the statue found a home in the back parking lot, safe from bus drivers, anarchists, radicals, etc. You can visit it by asking at the front desk—but check your bombs first.

day (an odd concept in this era of ladder-climbing face-time) but also was the spark for May Day as celebrated around the world. In this country capitalists were successful in getting the day redefined as the domain of socialists and communists.

● Walk two blocks south to the corner of W. Madison St. and N. Des Plaines Ave. An outgrowth of the government reforms decried by many conservatives as socialist today, the Social Security Administration Building (later renamed for Harold Washington) is as gray a government edifice as you'd expect. Fun, however, comes from the huge *Bat Column* sculpture by Claes Oldenburg.

- Cross the Madison St. Bridge over the expressway and stop at the corner of Halsted St. In 1949 photographer Art Shay took an iconic photo of author Nelson Algren standing on this corner flanked by a woman of flexible morals and a man seconds away from passing out. You can smell the skid marks of skid row, and this was the milieu that Algren recorded in books like *The Man With the Golden Arm*. Today you're likely to be in shadow from glossy developments like Skybridge on the northeast corner.

- Turn south down S. Halsted St. This is the heart of Greektown, home of what was once the city's main Greek community. Almost eradicated by the expressway in the 1960s, it hung on thanks in no small part to hunks of flaming cheese called "saganaki." Various crowd-pleasing, often-uproarious Greek restaurants like the Parthenon (314 S. Halsted St.), where saganaki was invented, kept lines forming even as the surrounding blocks died. Today there's still a definite Greek accent here. Among the highlights on S. Halsted: the Hellenic Museum (southwest corner of W. Adams St., although a new location is in the offing), which traces the experience of immigrants who at one time operated most of the coffee shops in Chicago; the Athenian Candle Company (300), which still dips its own candles; the Artopolis Bakery Cafe Agora (306), an upscale place for a tiny cup of strong coffee; the Pan Hellenic Pastry Shop (324), where you won't escape not sticky from baklava; and Athens Grocery (324), which is the place to buy some cheap ouzo for lighting up your own cheese—and liver.

- Head west on W. Van Buren St. and turn south on S. Morgan St. Go one block and stop at the northwest corner of S. Tilden St. This otherwise humdrum building was once the warehouse for the Reliance Corporation. Now it is notable for the extravagant 1984 mural by Richard Haas on its south and west sides. Among the highlights is a segment depicting Daniel Burnham's unrealized 1909 plan for a grand civic center that would have been based here. Use the Morgan St. bridge over the Eisenhower Expressway for the best vantage.

- Tilden ends at S. Aberdeen St. Go two blocks north to W. Jackson Blvd. and turn west. The striking façade on the Hubbard St. Dance Centre (1147) shows how far this company has come—literally and figuratively—since its founding by the legendary Lou Conte in 1977. Studios here host classes and performances (main stage works are at the Harris Theater in Millennium Park).

- Continue west on Jackson Blvd. Passing S. Throop St., you'll see the Chicago Police Training Center on the north side of the street. There are often gaggles of fresh-faced recruits doing calisthenics outside. This is not the time to wander over and offer a bribe. West of S. Laflin St. the 1500 block of Jackson was a stylish island in the 1880s (this area was otherwise given over to sweatshops, slums and bawdyhouses). With its huge oaks arching over the street and numerous preserved homes, it is a seductive mixture of Second Empire, Italianate, Queen Anne and other styles. Of note are homes at 1501, 1506, 1531 and 1532.

- Turn north one block on busy S. Ashland Ave. The crowds often seen at 204 are there for the Mexican Consulate.

- At W. Adams St, walk east for one block. The Church of the Epiphany (1885) on the southeast corner is a rich riot of carved stone. The lovely home at 1535 is an early example (1874) of what could be accomplished with Joliet limestone.

- At S. Laflin St., walk north two blocks, and take the jog slightly east on W. Madison St. as it becomes N. Bishop St. Go one block north to W. Washington Blvd., then jog west 150 feet to N. Ogden Ave. Go northeast one block to W. Randolph St. On your west, Union Park dates from 1853. Look for the statue of Carter H. Harrison, a mayor in the late 1800s whose relentless boosterism earned Chicago the moniker "Windy City" (and not because of excessive sauerkraut consumption as some Brits suppose). His assassination by a job-seeker in 1893 ended the Columbian Exposition on a sour note.

- Head east on W. Randolph St. This triple boulevard has been given a real spiffing up in recent years. Always home to light industry, it is a center of media and restaurant supply companies. At 1313, look for the flowers on the 1928 Art Deco warehouse that was once a flower market.

- Turn south one block on N. Aberdeen St. and continue east on W. Washington Blvd. If you see lots of people clutching copies of, say, *A Million Little Lies*, er, I mean *Pieces* by James Frey, you will know immediately you've found Harpo Studios, production home of book-club maven and billionaire broadcaster Oprah Winfrey. On weekdays there's bodacious hordes of people waiting to be in the audience.

At the southwest corner of N. Morgan St., Wishbone is always packed with fans both of Oprah and the fab southern food. (Bring on the corn muffins!)

- Walk north on N. Morgan St. As you cross Randolph, you're in the heart of the restaurant supply district. On the south side of the street you can load up on 10,000 paper napkins; on the north look for cans of food in quantities that make Costco seem like a 7-11. (If you need a more manageable bite, try the classic dogs at Market St. Inn.) Two blocks farther on at Fulton Market, you are in the heart of the heart of the wholesale food market. Come pre-dawn for the greatest action. Later in the day, you're less likely to get knocked upside the head by a gross of kumquats, and instead can appreciate the many galleries that are supplanting the food suppliers. The 1000 block of W. Fulton St. is especially chock-a-block.

- Walk east on Fulton to N. Halsted St. and turn north, crossing the long, barren bridge. Below, Chicago's transport legacy is in full view, from the underground Kennedy Expressway to mainline railroad tracks that see Amtrak trains going as far as Seattle. Cross under yet more tracks (Metra to suburbs galore) and turn east to the relative quiet of W. Hubbard St.

- Make a sharp turn northwest on N. Milwaukee Ave. Look for the book-cluttered window at 459. N. Fagin Books is one of Chicago's unheralded gems of a used bookstore. This is the place to find rare tomes on anthropology, zoology, botany and more. It's a creationist's nightmare.

- End your walk at the six corners of Milwaukee, Halsted and W. Grand Ave. Depending on your tastes, there's fun in all directions. If it's after 10 PM, just

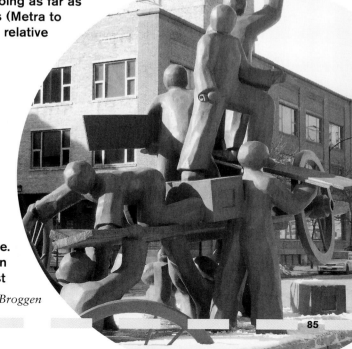

Haymarket sculpture by Mary Broggen

east is Funky Buddha Lounge, an eclectic joint for R&B, House, Disco and more. Just north, Doolin's is the place for rubber chickens, Three Stooges props, helium for balloons or voice high-jinks and pretty much anything else you might want for a party. When it's time to go, the Blue Line El Grand station is just below.

POINTS OF INTEREST

Parthenon 314 S. Halsted St., 312-726-2407

Athenian Candle Company 300 S. Halsted St., 312-332-6988

Artopolis Bakery Cafe Agora 306 S. Halsted St., 312-559-9000

Pan Hellenic Pastry Shop 324 S. Halsted St., 312-454-1886

Athens Grocery 324 S. Halsted St., 312-454-0940

Hubbard St. Dance Centre www.hubbardstreetdance.org, 1147 W. Jackson Blvd., 312-850-9744

Wishbone 1001 W. Washington Blvd., 312-850-2663

Market St. Inn 955 W. Randolph St., 312-829-9170

N. Fagin Books 459 N. Milwaukee Ave., 312-829-5252

Funky Buddha 728 W. Grand Ave., 312-666-1695

Doolin's 511 N. Halsted St., 312-243-9424

route summary

1. Start at the intersection of W. Randolph St. and N. Des Plaines Ave.
2. Walk two blocks south to the corner of W. Madison St. and N. Des Plaines Ave.
3. Cross the Madison St. Bridge.
4. Turn left down S. Halsted St.
5. Turn right on W. Van Buren St.
6. Turn left on S. Morgan St. Go one block and stop at the northwest corner of S. Tilden St.
7. Go right on Tilden, which ends at S. Aberdeen St.

8. Go two blocks north on S. Aberdeen.

9. Turn left on W. Jackson Blvd.

10. Turn right one block on S. Ashland Ave.

11. At W. Adams St, turn right and walk east for one block.

12. At S. Laflin St., turn left and walk north two blocks, and take the jog slightly east on W. Madison St. as it becomes N. Bishop St.

13. Go one block north to W. Washington Blvd., jog left 150 feet to N. Ogden Ave.

14. Turn right and go northeast one block to W. Randolph St.

15. Turn right on W. Randolph St.

16. Turn right on N. Aberdeen St. and go south one block.

17. Turn left east on W. Washington Blvd.

18. Turn left on N. Morgan St.

19. Turn right on W. Fulton St.

20. Turn left on N. Halsted St., crossing the long bridge.

21. Turn right to W. Hubbard St.

22. Make a sharp left turn northwest on N. Milwaukee Ave.

23. End your walk at the six corners of Milwaukee, Halsted and W. Grand Ave.

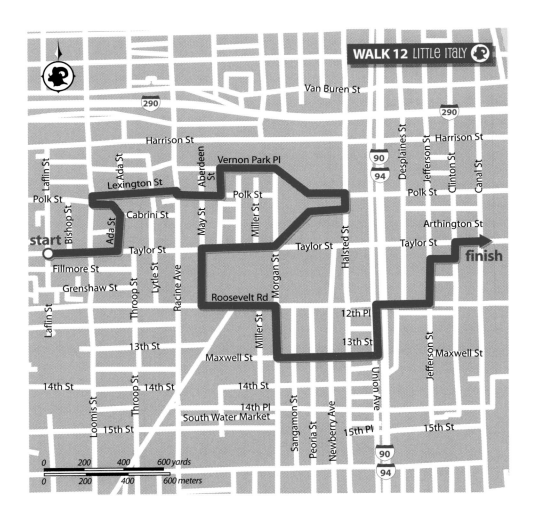

Van Buren St

290

Harrison St

Vernon Park Pl

290

Desplaines St

Harrison St

Jefferson St

Clinton St

Canal St

90

94

Laflin St

Ada St

Lexington St

Polk St

Bishop St

Ada St

Cabrini St

Aberdeen St

May St

Miller St

Polk St

Polk St

start

Taylor St

Fillmore St

Grenshaw St

Throop St

Lytle St

Racine Ave

Taylor St

Halsted St

Arthington St

Taylor St

finish

Laflin St

13th St

Roosevelt Rd

Morgan St

Maxwell St

12th Pl

13th St

Jefferson St

Maxwell St

14th St

Throop St

14th St

Loomis St

15th St

Maxwell St

Miller St

14th St

14th Pl

South Water Market

Sangamon St

Peoria St

Newberry Ave

Union Ave

13th St

15th Pl

90

94

15th St

0   200   400   600 yards

0   200   400   600 meters

12 LITTLE ITaLY: SURVIVAL OF THE FITTEST

BOUNDARIES: **W. Harrison St., S. Canal St., W. Maxwell St., S. Ashland Ave.**
DISTANCE: **3.3 miles**
PUBLIC TRANSIT: **9 Ashland and 12 Roosevelt Busses**

Little Italy was never populated exclusively by Italians. In fact the Irish were the majority for many years. But along the commercial hub of Taylor St. it was the Italians who owned the shops and restaurants, giving the neighborhood its enduring ethnic feel. Long a tidy enclave close to the Loop, Little Italy suffered from a lack of clout with the Irish mafia that ran Chicago. In the late 1930s, a huge public housing development split the community in two. In the 1950s expressway construction destroyed thousands of homes and hemmed in the survivors. Then in the 1960s the construction of a new university destroyed hundreds more. Still the neighborhood hung on, and today it is thriving. West of Ashland, medical schools and hospitals contribute scores of residents (no pun intended). New condos of the usual highly variable quality are springing up between shady blocks of sturdy two-flats and long-running Italian businesses. Only the recent wanton destruction of the Maxwell St. Market shows that some things never change.

- Start your walk in the old Little Italy neighborhood at the corner of W. Taylor St. and S. Laflin St. The original Rosebud is on the northwest corner and has been one of the city's classic Italian restaurants for over 30 years. Named after the native flower of Sicily, it's one of the few places in town to boast a photo of Frank Sinatra that was actually taken here. Note that, should you lunch here, you may need bearers to carry your over-stuffed hulk for the rest of the walk.

- Walk east on Taylor, enjoying the relaxed tree-lined feel. At Chirugi Hardware (1449), there are toilet seats in the window, but it's what comes first that's important, a vast selection of wine-making gear; at Conte Di Savoia (1438), amidst the intoxicating aromas of Tuscany there is an entire row of olive oils.

- Stop at Piazza DiMaggio, a rather curious public space in that it's named for Joe DiMaggio, the proud son of San Francisco whose only Chicago connection was being turned down by the Chicago Cubs (probably a career benefit). But turn and face south and a dim explanation appears: the National Italian American Sports Hall of Fame, a well-funded center that's just what the name implies.

- Continuing east on Taylor, only the pure won't stop at Scafuri Bakery, where for over 100 years the same family has been making luscious cannoli.

- At S. Ada St., turn north. Notice the decayed building on the northeast corner, all that remains of the Jane Addams Homes, the first federally-subsidized housing project in Chicago. It opened in 1938 to great acclaim and closed in 2002 after it had become an insult to its namesake (see later in walk) through mismanagement and anemic funding. The section you see here is all that remains of the vast complex that divided Little Italy. It is intended to someday open as a Public Housing Museum. Meantime upscale homes of every kind are going up at a rapid rate.

- Cut northwest across leafy Arrigo Park until you see the looming statue of Columbus near S. Loomis St. Many think he looks like Victor Mature of *The Robe* era.

- Walk across the park northeast to W. Lexington St. At 1254, you'll find some of Chicago's oldest homes, five rowhouses dating from the mid-1870s. Built when this was a tiny Irish enclave, note how large blocks have been carved to resemble smaller stones—sort of the Z-brick of its day. A bit farther, the 1911 Shrine of Our Lady of Pompeii was saved from closing by the Archdiocese in 1985 by wily parishioners, who had the church redesignated as a shrine staffed by their own order of priests.

- Continue east and then jog down S. Racine Ave. slightly to W. Polk St. These bucolic streets are one of the reasons that Little Italy hung on after World War II and is thriving again. At S. Aberdeen St. turn north past two alleys and saunter through the charming little pedestrian area to W. Vernon Park Pl. On your right is one of Little Italy's most charming family-run restaurants, Tufano's Vernon Park Tap.

- Head east on Vernon Park until the street ends at a turn-around. You are now at the northwest corner of the University of Illinois at Chicago. When it opened in 1965 it was a dramatic statement by architect Walter Netsch, who proclaimed a visit to the campus akin to exploring a Tuscan hill town. Well, maybe after the apocalypse, as Netsch's love of Brutalism was on full display. Raised walkways traversed the campus, leaving the ground-level to rats and students diving into Dumpsters for exam answers. Beginning in the 1990s, the details of Netsch's "village" were demolished to leave the far more pedestrian-friendly campus you see here—although excesses in concrete remain controversial. From your entry at the end of Vernon Park Pl., look north to the hive-like Behavioral Sciences Building (1967), the source of perennial jokes about rats, cheese and mazes. Right ahead, the 28-story University Hall (1965) housed faculty and administrators who could peer down on students navigating their own maze of the original campus.

- Walk southeast across campus to the enticingly named Campus Core, which is actually a good common area with plenty of benches and places for snacks. Originally a commuter school, UIC is busily adding dorms for its 25,000 students; many line S. Halsted St. to the east.

- Walk east and through the humdrum Student Center East to Halsted and turn south. Immediately on your right is one of two surviving buildings of the Jane Addams Hull House. Dating from 1856, the heavily reconstructed wood-frame structure is now a museum of Addams and her organization, which served thousands of impoverished immigrants in the area beginning in 1889. The 13-structure campus had bathhouses, medical facilities, schools, galleries, kitchens and much more. The one surviving building is the Dining Hall (1905), just south of the museum. Through the 1960s, the organization espoused the belief that immigrants were worth far more than the puny value attached to them by exploitive employers.

- Just south of the Dining Hall, cut diagonally southwest across campus to the corner of S. Morgan St. and W. Taylor St.

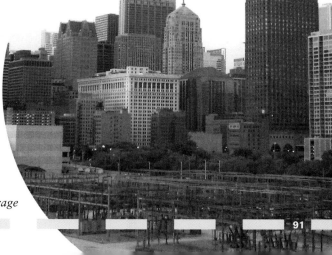

View from the new Whole Foods parking garage

- Walk west on Taylor, looking for the following highlights which give this bit of Little Italy a more blue-collar feel: at Nea Agora (1056) lamb's the specialty, and you'll see whole ones (sans innards, ick) going out the door on the shoulders of employees; Mario's Italian Lemonade (1068), home of fresh-squeezed summertime joy; and Al's No. 1 Italian Beef (1079), a spot that sparks many an argument among local Italian beef lovers.

- Turn south on S. May St. and walk through a few pedestrian zones to busy W. Roosevelt Rd. Immediately to your left is the massive Holy Family Church, an institution as unbowed as its Jesuit patrons. It dates from 1857. Next door is the imposing bulk of St. Ignatius College Prep, the clout-heavy school whose notable grads include local luminaries (Bob Newhart graduated from here in 1947). Stroll the gardens, which feature many an architectural artifact from demolished local masterpieces, including a horny one from the Chicago Herald building.

- A long block east, cross south on S. Morgan St. one block to the northwest corner of W. Maxwell St. Listen for the sound of a garage door rolling up, followed by the moody refrain of Mike Post's theme song. Recognize this building? In its former life as a grungy Chicago police station, it was the opening credits icon of *Hill Street Blues*, the landmark drama that ran from 1981 to 1987. The series never was specifically based in Chicago (just a similarly gritty city) and it was actually filmed in Los Angeles. Before UIC cleaned it up for its own force, Chicago cops called this place home from 1888 to 1998.

- Walk east on W. Maxwell St., through the section that's just sidewalk between ballfields, and then again on the street until you reach S. Halsted St. Try not to break down and cry. This was ground zero of the old Maxwell Street Market, the chaotic and legendary open-air bazaar that lasted for a hundred years until the early 1990s. Generations of immigrants sold everything from screws to cheap suits (extra pair of pants free!). The air was redolent with the smells of classic Chicago pork chop sandwiches, while some of the first legendary blues musicians played on the streets for nickels. Today what you see is simply a travesty of bland gentrification, right down to the Jamba Juice (a Jamba Juice!!!).

- Hurriedly cut through the building built over Maxwell St. east to narrow S. Union St. hard by the expressway. Head north and follow your nose like a grease-seeking dog to Jim's, the "relocated" landmark that once stood where Jamba Juice is now located. Chomp into a pork chop sandwich or knock back a Polish sausage while enjoying the cheap prices and free fries. Note that the street gets jammed with everything from double-parked delivery vans to Cadillacs at lunch.

- Continue north on Union St. to Roosevelt Rd. and turn east, crossing the noxious Dan Ryan Expressway. At S. Jefferson St. turn north. Immediately on the east side of the street, you'll see mobs of cars triple-parked in front of Manny's. Lovers of pastrami, potato pancakes and other classic deli items reach a state of bliss—and future coronary failure—at this institution.

- One street past Manny's, on the east side of Jefferson, look for a bland 1960s government building with a bronze flame out front. This is the Chicago Fire Academy, which with ham-fisted irony is built on the site of the start of the 1871 Chicago fire. Although a cow belonging to Mrs. O'Leary long took the blame for the udder destruction of what was then America's fourth-largest city, recent research points elsewhere. It seems O'Leary had rented out her barn to a certain Daniel "Peg Leg" Sullivan, who was not very stable on his, er, foot. After knocking over a lantern, the panicked Sullivan blamed the bovine. In 1997 the Chicago City Counsel officially absolved the cow.

- Walk east across parking lot south of the academy—which was once W. De Koven St.—then turn north on S. Clinton St. and take an immediate right on W. Taylor St. one block to S. Canal St. Looming in front of you is the latest big-box invader of the South Loop. Take the plunge inside—avoiding the siren song of a studded dog collar at Pet Smart or the allure of one of 157 varieties of rice milk at Whole Foods—and take the elevator to the top floor of the parking garage. Here, amidst happy shoppers loading their trunks with organic toast, you can marvel at the sweeping views in all directions. Just north, the Sears Tower looms large. Looking west at sunset, you can see the red glow behind the steeples of Holy Family Church.

- From here walk 0.6 of a mile east on the Roosevelt Ave. Bridge to the Red, Green and Orange Lines El stop at Roosevelt, or use the 12 Roosevelt Bus.

CONNECTING THE WALKS

From the El stop you can connect to Walks 13 and 23.

POINTS OF INTEREST

Rosebud 1550 W. Taylor St., 312-755-1777

National Italian American Sports Hall of Fame 1431 W. Taylor St., 312-226-5566

Chirugi Hardware 1449 W. Taylor St., 312-666-2235

Conte Di Savoia 1438 W. Taylor St., 312-666-3471

Scafuri Bakery 1337 W. Taylor St., 312-733-8881

Tufano's Vernon Park Tap 1073 W. Vernon Park Pl., 312-733-3393

University of Illinois at Chicago www.uic.edu, 312-996-7000

Jane Addams Hull House Museum 800 S. Halsted St, 312-413-5353

Nea Agora 1056 W. Taylor St., 312-271-2080

Mario's Italian Lemonade 1068 W. Taylor St.

Al's No. 1 Italian Beef 1079 W. Taylor St., 312-226-4017

Jim's 1250 S. Union Ave., 312-733-7820

Manny's 1141 S. Jefferson St., 312-939-2855

ROUTE SUMMARY

1. Start at the corner of W. Taylor St. and S. Laflin St.
2. Walk east on Taylor.
3. At S. Ada St., turn left.
4. Cut northwest across Arrigo Park to the statue of Columbus near S. Loomis St.
5. Walk across the park northeast to W. Lexington St.
6. Continue east and then jog right down S. Racine Ave. to W. Polk St.
7. At S. Aberdeen St. turn left past two alleys to W. Vernon Park Pl.

8. Turn right on Vernon Park until the street ends at a turn-around.

9. Walk southeast across campus to the Campus Core.

10. Walk east and through the Student Center East to Halsted and turn right.

11. Just south of the Jane Addams Hull House Dining Hall, cut diagonally southwest across campus to the corner of S. Morgan St. and W. Taylor St.

12. Walk west on Taylor.

13. Turn south on S. May St. to W. Roosevelt Rd.

14. Walk a long block east.

15. Cross south on S. Morgan St. one block to the northwest corner of W. Maxwell St.

16. Walk east on W. Maxwell St., on the sidewalk between ballfields, and then again on the street until you reach S. Halsted St.

17. Cut through the building built over Maxwell St. going east to S. Union St.

18. Turn left on Union St. to Roosevelt Rd.

19. Turn right, crossing the Dan Ryan Expressway.

20. At S. Jefferson St. turn left.

21. Walk east across the parking lot south of the academy, then turn left on S. Clinton St.

22. Take an immediate right on W. Taylor St.

23. Walk one block to S. Canal St. and take the elevator to the top floor of the parking garage at Whole Foods.

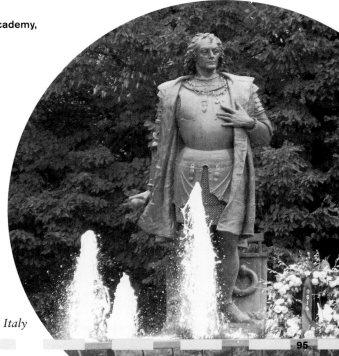

Columbus statue, Little Italy

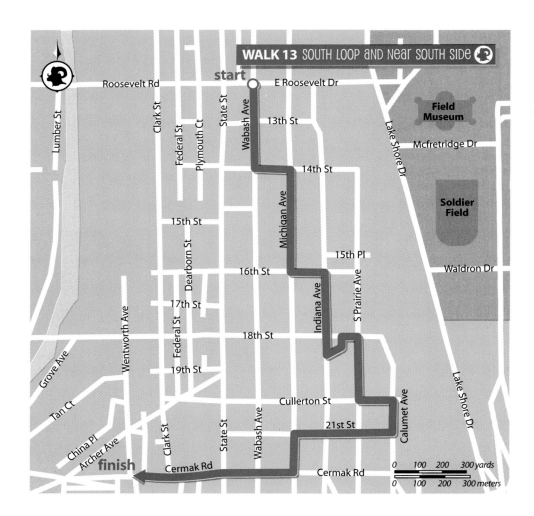

start

finish

Roosevelt Rd

E Roosevelt Dr

Field
Museum

Mcfretridge Dr

Soldier
Field

Waldron Dr

13th St

14th St

15th Pl

16th St

17th St

18th St

19th St

Cullerton St

21st St

Cermak Rd

Cermak Rd

15th St

Lumber St

Clark St

Federal St

Plymouth Ct

State St

Wabash Ave

Michigan Ave

Dearborn St

Wentworth Ave

Grove Ave

Tan Ct

China Pl

Archer Ave

Clark St

Federal St

State St

Wabash Ave

Indiana Ave

S Prairie Ave

Calumet Ave

Lake Shore Dr

Lake Shore Dr

| 0 | 100 | 200 | 300 yards |
| 0 | 100 | 200 | 300 meters |

13 SOUTH LOOP aND Near SOUTH SiDe: FrOM B-GirLS TO B-FLaTS

BOUNDARIES: E. Roosevelt Rd., S. Calumet Ave., E. 22nd St./W Cermak Rd., S. State St.
DISTANCE: 2 miles
PUBLIC TRANSIT: Green, Orange and Red Lines El to Roosevelt

Once hemmed in by railroads, the South Loop and Near South Side have a history as varied as any in the city. These were the first areas settled—somewhat disastrously—by whites, and later were home to Chicago's elite. Industry and vice came later, the latter in extraordinary proportions. Today the area is a fast-growing, upscale residential neighborhood that combines old and new buildings in ways that would surprise anyone who lived here in the past.

- Start your walk at the corner of W. Roosevelt Rd. and S. Wabash Ave. Everything you see around you is a consequence of Chicago's railroad legacy. Facing south, the huge tower looming to the east by the park is part of Central Station, a development over the old Illinois Central Railroad yards. It's named for the terminal that stood at the corner of Roosevelt and S. Michigan Ave., once the starting point for famous trains such as—cue Arlo Guthrie—the City of New Orleans. It was also the final destination for tens of thousands of southern blacks during the Great Migration in the early 20th century. To your right, the seemingly endless low- and mid-rise developments west of S. State St. are built on the site of the yards for the Santa Fe Railroad.

- Walk one block south on Wabash to E. 13th St. The sleek building on the southeast corner with the curving glass block front was once the film exchange building for Universal Pictures. (Although the yellow-brick façade might suggest MGM and the Yellow Brick Road.) This entire area in the 1930s was a distribution hub for the U.S. film industry. Copies of films moved by train, and it seemed every train stopped in Chicago. The studios operated these huge vaults as distribution centers for the country. Warner Bros. was just south at 1307, while Paramount was east of Universal at the southwest corner of 13th and S. Michigan Ave. (now a dance studio for Columbia College). Opera, the flamboyant Chinese restaurant in the Universal building, is an example of the many upscale eateries that opened around here in the last few years. In fact, some especially romantic tables are nestled in the old film vaults at Opera.

Continue south, go east one block on E. 14th St. to S. Michigan Ave. and turn south. Like the rest of the area, there's a mix of loft-conversions, residential rehabs and new high-rise condo towers along here. If you see people out undaunted by neither snow nor rain nor heat nor gloom of night, then they may be members of the National Association of Letter Carriers at 1411 S. Michigan.

● Walk under the Canadian National rail overpass just north of 16th St. (a still vital link for Great Plains grain headed for the Gulf Coast ports) and turn east on E. 16th St.

● Turn south on S. Indiana Ave. and continue until you reach E. 18th St. The next few blocks are filled with things to see. On the southeast corner, drop into the National Vietnam Veterans Art Museum. Originally a struggling place where vets could display their artworks during the early 1990s when the entire area was still two clicks above decrepit, the museum has developed into a nationally renowned venue that uses art and other exhibits to examine the effects of war. The works are perplexing, moving and stark; recent displays begin to address the invasion of Iraq.

● Just south, the Clark House is a contender for the oldest building in Chicago. Parts date back to 1836 when it was built a couple blocks away at 1700 S. Michigan Ave. Since it was moved to its present location, lavish gardens have been planted on the grounds. On a pretty day, you may want to take an extended pause, sitting in the shade under a tree, smelling the scents from the beds of wildflowers.

● From the gardens, take the exit north to E. 18th St. On your left is the Vietnam Veterans Art Museum, which also houses the truly splendid Cafe Society. The personable staff serve a range of casual meals you can enjoy at tables on the shady plaza.

● Walk east on 18th and notice the building on your right. Parents may want to protect the sensibilities of their children in case there are any architects present, as they tend to get all hot and bothered by the John J. Glessner House. Considered by many the finest structure in Chicago, this vision in pinkish granite was the work of Henry Hobson Richardson in 1885. On one of the frequent tours, you can appreciate the sheer luxury

Back Story: Fort Dearborn Massacre

Chicago in 1812 was little more than a fort named Dearborn near where the Michigan Ave. bridge today crosses the Chicago River. The area was alive with Indian tribes, many aligned with the British instead of the Americans. (Many others were aligned with John Kinzie, a trader and future street name, who profited from the sales of cheap booze.) On August 15, the garrison decided to flee Chicago with a large party of women and children. They got about two miles and were then surrounded and slaughtered by various tribes. More than 50 died, and as close as anybody can determine, it happened right at today's intersection of S. Prairie Ave. and E. 18th St. When he had a mansion there in the 1880s, rail baron George Pullman had a large memorial to the massacre on his property, but both are now long gone.

of the interior, right out of an English manor house. The south-facing courtyard may make you wish you could put in an offer now (and had a spare $20 million).

- Outside the Glessner House, stand at the intersection of 18th and S. Prairie Ave. and look south. In the 1880s, you would have seen the finest street in the city, with one gracious mansion giving way to another. In 1980, you would have seen virtual squalor, with a few surviving mansions in ratty shape amidst vast areas of rubble. Now this is ground zero for the rebirth of the Near South Side, and the stately rows of new homes blend in with restored gems from the past. Still, historic echoes are all around. (See the sidebar for details of the Fort Dearborn massacre.)

- Walk south on Prairie. Proof that politics, like love, is fickle can be found—or not found—just south of the Glessner House. While you do see the gardens of the Clark House, what you don't see is the Hillary Rodham Clinton Women's Park, which was announced with great fanfare by the city when the then-first lady visited town for her 50th birthday in 1997. As allegiances later shifted, the Daley administration simply forgot all about it.

- Look for excellent plaques along Prairie that give details of life in the neighborhood during the best of times and—you saw it coming—the worst of times. Stop at 1900, an

1870 mansion that managed to retain its dignity through the years and today is not as over-restored as some survivors. In fact, turn around and look at 1919. This 1884 mansion was the home of Marshall Field Jr., and was one of the finest on the block. (Field Jr. was not a chip off his famous father's block, and he died here in 1905 after a much-discussed afternoon in the Levee District, see below.) But by the 1930s it had become a rooming house, and by the 1980s it was a crack house. Today it comprises six condos (at close to $2 million each) and you'd be hard-pressed to deduce its original appearance.

- Turn east on E. Cullerton St. Amidst the new homes, you can see a few of the industrial buildings that dominated the area for much of the 20th century. Although the mansions of Prairie Avenue were built to last hundreds of years, the neighborhood wasn't. The Chicago fire caused a long-term shift of industry to the near south side. The good rail links only drew more industry, and by 1900, it was really ill-suited for millionaires, who fled their newish mansions for the Gold Coast and Kenwood.

- Head south on S. Calumet Ave., noting another surviving mansion (1870) at 2020. At the corner of E. 21st St., behold a virtual industrial cathedral stretching south for the southeast corner. Built over many years beginning in the 1920s, the R.R. Donnelley and Sons printing plant expressed every bit of pride they had in their business. For more than 50 years, a large number of America's magazines like *Life* and *Time* were printed here. Look at the exterior details that include medieval shields, finely carved stone balconies, low-hanging fruit in the form of grapes and much more. Today, rather fittingly, the presses are silent, but the complex is still in the media business as a server farm and vast datacenter for a variety of internet firms.

- Walk three blocks west on E. 21st St. to S. Michigan Ave. and turn south. Willie Dixon's Blues Heaven Foundation preserves the Chess Records building. Dixon began the foundation to preserve the legacy of the blues, work carried on by his daughter Shirli until her untimely death in 2003. But the foundation continues, and for blues fans, this is a shrine. The Chess Brothers—two Polish Jews—loved the blues and recorded the likes of Muddy Waters and Bo Diddley. The Rolling Stones made their own pilgrimage here in 1963 to record and learn the blues. They named an instrumental "2120 South Michigan Avenue" in honor of the place.

- At E. 22nd St. (Cermak Rd.), turn west and walk to the intersection with S. State St. Today you see the curvaceous charms of the Hilliard Homes, a former nasty public housing project that, in a sign of what's going on in the 'hood, has been rehabbed into upscale apartments. In 1900, however, the curvaceous charms here were of a different sort. North from 22nd and west of State was the notorious Levee District, one of the largest collections of whorehouses in the world. Hundreds of brothels, grand and humble, catered to every whim and budget. All this sex finally stimulated a reaction from officials (many of whom were regulars), and the Levee, including the infamous Everleigh Club, was shut down in 1912.

- Walk one block farther west to the Red Line El stop at Cermak-Chinatown.

CONNECTING THE WALKS

At the end of this walk you can join Walk 15 for Chinatown. You can also extend your walk at the start by linking up with Walk 23.

POINTS OF INTEREST

Opera 1301 S. Wabash Ave., 312-461-0161

National Vietnam Veterans Art Museum www.nvvam.org, 1801 S. Indiana Ave., 312-326-0270

Cafe Society 1801 S. Indiana Ave., 312-842-4210

John J. Glessner House www.glessnerhouse.org, 1800 S. Prairie Ave., 312-326-1480

Willie Dixon's Blues Heaven Foundation 2120 S. Michigan Ave., 312-808-1286

route summary

1. Start at the corner of W. Roosevelt Rd. and S. Wabash Ave.
2. Walk south on Wabash to E. 14th St.
3. Turn left and go east one block on E. 14th St. to S. Michigan Ave. then turn right.
4. Turn left on E. 16th St.
5. Turn right on S. Indiana Ave. and continue until you reach E. 18th St.
6. Enter the Clark House from S. Indiana Ave.
7. From the gardens, take the exit north to E. 18th St.
8. Walk east on 18th to S. Prairie Ave.
9. Turn right on Prairie.
10. Turn left on E. Cullerton St.
11. Turn right on S. Calumet Ave.
12. Turn right and walk three blocks west on E. 21st St. to S. Michigan Ave. then turn left.
13. At E. 22nd St. (Cermak Rd.), turn right and walk to the Red Line El stop at Cermak-Chinatown.

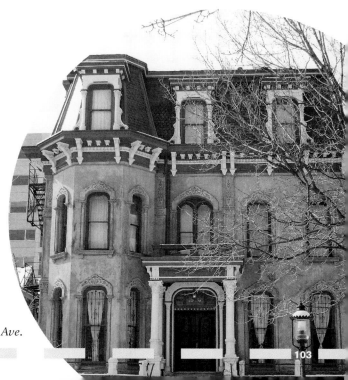

1900 S. Prairie Ave.

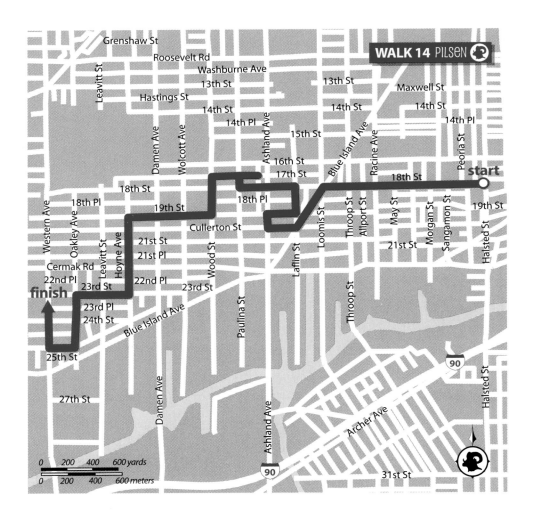

Grenshaw St

Roosevelt Rd

Washburne Ave

13th St

Hastings Ave

14th St

14th Pl

18th St

18th Pl

19th St

Cullerton St

21st St

21st Pl

22nd Pl

23rd St

13th St

14th St

15th St

16th St

17th St

Maxwell St

14th St

14th Pl

18th St

19th St

21st St

start

finish

Leavitt St

Damen Ave

Wolcott Ave

Ashland Ave

Blue Island Ave

Racine Ave

Peoria St

Halsted St

Western Ave

18th Pl

Oakley Ave

Leavitt St

Hoyne Ave

Wood St

Laflin St

Loomis St

Throop St

Allport St

May St

Morgan St

Sangamon St

Cermak Rd

22nd Pl

23rd St

22nd Pl

23rd St

23rd Pl

24th St

Blue Island Ave

Paulina St

Throop St

25th St

27th St

Damen Ave

Ashland Ave

Archer Ave

Halsted St

31st St

90

90

0   200   400   600 yards
0   200   400   600 meters

14 PILSEN: FROM BOHEMIA TO MEXICO TO BOHEMIAN

BOUNDARIES: W. 17th St., S. Halsted St., S. Blue Island Ave., S. Western Ave.
DISTANCE: 3.7 miles
PUBLIC TRANSIT: 8 Halsted bus

Beginning in the 1870s, scores of Bohemian immigrants filled the neighborhood that came to bear the sentimental moniker "Pilsen," for the city of the Central European homeland. Huge factories consumed the labors of thousands of unskilled workers, and exploitation made Pilsen a hotbed of the labor movement. Meanwhile the mix of immigrants—Poland, Germany and Ireland were also represented here—got busy building some of Chicago's most dramatic churches. Early Mexican immigrants to Chicago found a home here in the 1930s. They gradually came to dominate the neighborhood, as you'll see from the myriad striking murals painted on the sides of the sturdy, brick buildings that still emit a Central European air. Today Bohemians are returning to Pilsen, although these are the kind who in cartoons munch brie and don black berets. The mix of artists and Hispanic culture has made Pilsen one of the most vibrant communities in the city.

- Give your walk a sweet start at Kristoffer's Cafe and Bakery right where W. 18th St. runs into S. Halsted St. Let the fabulous flan cakes envelop your tongue while you luxuriate on one of the couches. Emerging into the harsh realities of day, note that this bit of Halsted has a distinctly gentrified air. Just south, for God's sake, there's a yacht designer, and there are numerous galleries in a one-block radius. EXP Gallery around the corner on 18th St. east of Halsted is a prime example of the commitment here to local artists and contributes a modern-day Bohemian air.

- Begin your promenade west on 18th St. The street is lined with a mixture of sturdy vintage two- and three-flats, many of which have been gentrified with a Hispanic accent. But there are lots of other fill-in buildings, some unfortunately reaching a greedy four stories. A new flat in one of these averages $300,000, a bargain compared to the North Side.

● Continue west. Street vendors peddle treats throughout Pilsen, including the ever-popular slices of pineapple (*piña*) seasoned with special salt, or spicy cobs of corn (*elote*) dipped in butter. For something warmer, pop into Del Rey Tortilleria (1023) for a tortilla fresh from the ovens in back. In the next block, past S. Carpenter St., stop in front of 1125 and look for the carving that reads "Morticians" over the door. Across the street at 1140, there's a Romanesque gem of a four-flat. At the northeast corner of S. Allport St., St. Procopius Church continues the Romanesque theme (and there's more just north on Thalia Hall). Built in 1883, today it has masses in English, Spanish and Croatian. Murals can be found throughout Pilsen; those at the northeast corner of S. Throop St. are especially pious.

● Turn southwest on S. Blue Island Ave. More raggedy than 18th St., this commercial strip features the modern Pilsen logo of an eagle with a snake and a cactus in statue and silhouette. Among the surviving vintage buildings, look for the appropriately Pilsner connection at 1870, a once-Schlitz-brewery-owned corner tap.

● Go west on W. Cullerton St. The 1500 block here is a Pilsen classic: parked vans in various states of repair, Mexican music playing behind curtained windows, neighbors stoop-sitting and plastic flowers ringing the base of trees. The house at 1530 is typical of the late-1880s flats common in Pilsen. Take a moment to note how most houses on this walk have large gaps between their façades and the sidewalk. This is a legacy of the city's old street level, which wasn't much higher than the swamplands the city was built on. As a consequence, sewers were a mere fantasy and the reality was much nastier. By raising the streets (from four to 14 feet depending on the area), it was possible to get the nastiness to go down the drain. In Pilsen and other old neighborhoods, scores of houses built before the streets were raised aren't sure which floor is their main one.

● Turn north on S. Ashland Ave., where the blaring trucks will have you seeking shelter in less than a block at St. Pius V Church, at the southeast corner with W. 19th St. Masses at this fine example of Romanesque Revival (1885) are said in English and Spanish. If it all seems rather hopeless, join the dozens of others inside on daily pilgrimage to the rather famous Shrine of St. Jude, the patron saint of lost causes.

- Go east one block on 19th St. and then north two blocks on S. Laflin St. Turn west again on 18th St. These blocks have an enticing mix of classic restaurants, humble shops selling multiple variations on the Virgin Mary, trendy cafes and colorful galleries. BomBon Bakery (1508) is a local sensation, with owners who are protégés of Frontera Grill's Rick Bayless. The ever-expanding Restaurante Nuevo Leon (1515) is an anchor and boasts flamboyant murals inside and out. Artesanias D' Mexico (1644) is the place for Day of the Dead statues. Next door, Cafe Mestizo has coffee and open-mike nights for post-caffeinated local muses.

- Avoid the blight of the defunct gas station at the corner with S. Paulina St. and turn north one block to W. 17th St. and turn east again. The 185-foot terra-cotta towers on St. Adalbert Church cast shadows like those of a sundial. In fact, the passage of time here is all too apparent, as the church is showing the decades since 1915 when it was the pride of the local Polish community. The mostly unrestored workers' cottages on this block remain humble in the face of God.

- Walk west on 17th St. to S. Wood St. The roar of the El is overhead, and to the north are the busy Metra/BNSF tracks, with trains hauling commuters home and containers filled with imported goods that will soon join them.

- Go south on Wood past Harrison Park to W. 19th St. Lively anytime the temperature cracks 50, the park is Pilsen's floor show. Vendor carts surround the playground at the southwest corner. On warm evenings, a multi-cultural mix of kids attest to the vibrant ethnic dynamic of the neighborhood, and would surely bring a tear to the eye of an urban planner.

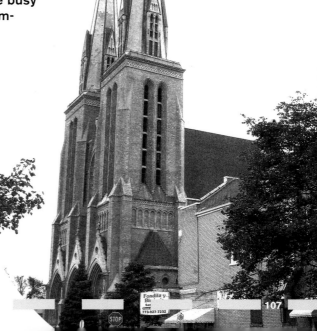

St. Paul's Church

- Go west along the south side of the park on 19th St. Midway, the National Museum of Mexican Art fills the old swimming pool building and modern additions. Works range from the historical to the modern, from Olmec carvings to Frida Kahlo drawings. West of the museum, baseball diamonds see some of Chicago's league soccer action on weekends.

- Cross busy S. Damen Ave. for the somewhat gentrified 2000 block of W. 19th St. It's all rather pleasant, and the odd plastic burro keeps things honest.

- Turn south on S. Hoyne Ave. and go 1.5 blocks to the west entrance to the El station. If you have an El pass or feel like you can part with the cost of a fare, enter and go up to the platform for sweeping views of Pilsen right to the Loop. The spires of churches such as St. Adalbert's and St. Paul's (see below) bear witness to a time when it was spiritual pursuits rather than the commercial that drove men toward the heavens.

- Just south of the El tracks, St. Matthew Lutheran Church plays an important role in the sanctuary movement, giving refugees support to flee conditions in their homelands. Note that St Matthäus is carved over the doors, an artifact of 1888 when parishioners all spoke German. Directly across W. 21st St. is the church's former school, one of Chicago's oldest schools (1882). Note the cute little cupola at the roof's apex.

- Continuing south, stop at the northwest corner with W. Cermak St. and look at the murals. Among the messages in a variety of languages is GLOBAL WARMING = GLOBAL WARNING, along with an image sure to gladden the heart of any CTA honcho: a rainbow leading from a dirty SUV to a bright and cheery bus.

- One block south of Cermak at W. 22nd Pl. is one of Chicago's loveliest churches. The twin steeples of St. Paul's soar 245 feet, and when new in 1897 were taller than anything in the Loop. Built with the hard-earned dimes of working-class parishioners, it is modeled on St. Cortin Cathedral in Normandy. The interior's Gothic beauty matches the exterior.

- Walk west two blocks on W. 23rd St. to S. Oakley Ave. Amidst the Bohemian heritage and Hispanic reality of Pilsen, a few blocks here in Oakley are resolutely Italian.

Home to a clutch of veteran restaurants that are constantly being "discovered" by new flocks of diners, S. Oakley has been beautified with fancy lamp posts and flowers south to W. Coulter St. (which is not named for the deranged commentator). La Fontanella (2414) has tables out front amidst flowers, while inside the flower of the neighborhood knocks back gulpable red at the bar. Just south, Bruna's Ristorante (2424) has classics like eggplant Parmigiana that date back to its opening in 1933. Or just follow your nose to the heady smells at Miceli's Deli (2448), which does sandwiches.

● Finish out Pilsen with a stroll to dusty and busy Western Ave. At the northeast corner of W. 23rd Pl., Donald's Hot Dogs serves up truly superlative Chicago-style dogs with an array of classic toppings. The humble aspirations of the menu are countered by the grand efforts in the kitchen.

● Take the 49 Western bus north to connections with the Blue and Orange Lines El.

POINTS OF INTEREST

Kristoffer's Cafe and Bakery 1733 S. Halsted St., 312-829-4150

EXP Gallery 726 W. 18th St., 847-217-7520

Del Rey Tortilleria 1023 W. 18th St., 312-829-3725

BomBon Bakery 1508 W. 18th St., 312-733-7788

Restaurante Nuevo Leon 1515 W. 18th St., 312-421-1517

Artesanias D' Mexico 1644 W. 18th St., 312-563-9779

Cafe Mestizo 1646 W. 18th St., 312-421-5920

La Fontanella 2414 S. Oakley Ave., 773-927-5249

Bruna's Ristorante 2424 S. Oakley Ave., 773-254-5550

Miceli's Deli 2448 S. Oakley Ave., 773-847-6873

Donald's Hot Dogs 2325 S. Western Ave., 773-254-7777

route summary

1. Start where W. 18th St. runs into S. Halsted St.
2. Go west on 18th St.
3. Turn left (southwest) on S. Blue Island Ave.
4. Turn right on W. Cullerton St.
5. Turn right on S. Ashland Ave.
6. Go east one block on W. 19th St.
7. Turn left and go north two blocks on S. Laflin St.
8. Turn left on 18th St.
9. Turn right one block on S. Paulina St. to W. 17th St.
10. Turn right and walk one half of a block.
11. Walk back west on 17th St. to S. Wood St.
12. Turn left on Wood; walk past Harrison Park to W. 19th St.
13. Turn right and walk along the south side of the park on 19th St.
14. Turn left on S. Hoyne Ave. and go 1½ blocks to the west entrance to the El station.
15. Continue south on Hoyne.
16. Turn right and walk west two blocks on W. 23rd St. to S. Oakley Ave.
17. Turn left on Oakley and walk south as far as W. 24th St..
18. Turn right on W. 23rd Pl. and walk west to S. Western Ave.

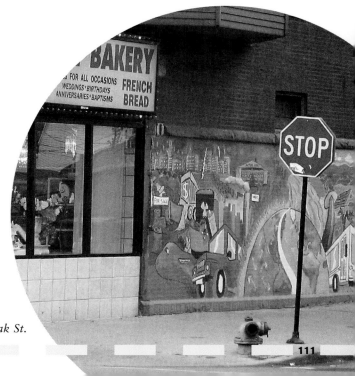

Colorful murals on W. Cermak St.

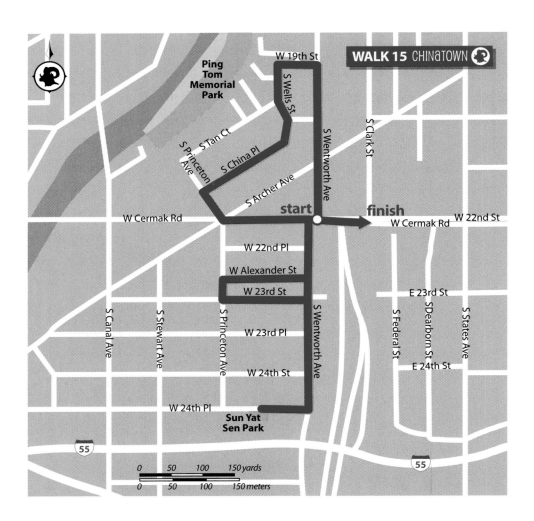

Ping
Tom
Memorial
Park

W 19th St

S Wells St

S Clark St

S Tan Ct

S China Pl

S Princeton Ave

S Archer Ave

S Wentworth Ave

W Cermak Rd

start

finish

W Cermak Rd

W 22nd St

W 22nd Pl

W Alexander St

W 23rd St

E 23rd St

S Canal Ave

S Stewart Ave

S Princeton Ave

W 23rd Pl

S Wentworth Ave

S Federal St

S Dearborn St

S States Ave

W 24th St

E 24th St

W 24th Pl

Sun Yat
Sen Park

55

55

0   50   100   150 yards

0   50   100   150 meters

15 CHINATOWN: WALKING WITH LIONS

BOUNDARIES: Chicago River South Branch, S. Wentworth Ave., W. 24th Pl., S. Princeton Ave.
DISTANCE: 2 miles
PUBLIC TRANSIT: Red Line El Cermak-Chinatown stop

For years a world unto itself, Chinatown has broken the shackles of expressways and railroads and is expanding to nearby South Side areas. Yet S. Wentworth Ave. remains the focus, and a trip here is like a little jaunt to Asia. There are shops and restaurants aimed at visitors, but most of daily life here revolves around commerce as new immigrants arrive daily. In the north, a spectacular new park along the river provides much-needed breathing room and a chance to join in the large groups stretching and exercising in the mornings.

● Start your walk facing the Chinese Gate over S. Wentworth Ave. It is an effective scene-setter and has an inscription that reads: THE WORLD BELONGS TO THE COMMONWEALTH, which loosely translated means "the common good," not the collection of former British colonies.

● Walk south on Wentworth. You will notice that the architecture here is an odd melange of traditional old Chicago—sturdy two- and three-story brick buildings—along with a smattering of structures that are much more clearly Chinese in inspiration. Many of the older structures have been given a thin veneer of "Chinese," such as pairs of ceramic evil-spirit-enemy lions. This reflects the fact that prior to 1910, this area was another Chicago neighborhood. After that date Chicago's Chinese coalesced in today's Chinatown, many fleeing rapidly rising rents in an older Chinatown in the Loop near today's Sears Tower.

● Stop in front of Pui Tak Center, the no-excuses Chinese building just south of the gate at 2216 S. Wentworth. Originally called the On Leong Building, it was built in 1928 by a Chinese merchant's association that found American architects who could "do" Chinese. Chicago's favorite architectural detail of the time, terra-cotta tiles, proved an able substitute for traditional Chinese glazed tiles. The building still serves as an important community center and landing spot for new arrivals looking for leads on jobs, housing and services. Through the years, the building has also starred in some spectacular raids by law enforcement types looking for gambling dens, organized crime and other vices.

- Continuing down Wentworth, you'll notice groups of Chinese, usually men, waiting in groups to be picked up by vans. These new arrivals are shuttled off to jobs at businesses run by established members of the community across the city. Although today's Chinatown is quite a vibrant community (it has spilled over its traditional boundaries south and west into Bridgeport and beyond), there are still a few businesses that milk the old clichés. Two restaurants opposite each other just south of W. 22nd Pl., Won Kow and Emperor's Choice, are classics. The former dates from 1927 and features a menu that is highlighted by such paper-umbrella drinks as mai-tais (served volcano-style, no less) at very cheap prices. At the latter, you enter past a rather grand façade and enjoy a menu that features dishes familiar to anyone who's ever read a Chung King label: egg foo yung and chop suey.

- The next few blocks are lined with some classic Chinese businesses. Look for groceries, noodle shops, boutiques and more. Many places have live fish swimming in the windows, awaiting their final role in a ceremonial dinner. Some highlights: Chiu Quon Bakery and Cafe (2242) has cases of treats including the best bargain locally, ham-filled buns for 75¢; Ten Ren Tea and Ginseng (2247), which has hundreds of bulk teas on display, some costing upwards of $139 a pound; Sun Sun Tong (2260), which has herbs and ginseng to cure maladies, although with many products having names like "Vigor" and "All Night Long," aging men would seem to be the target audience; and Hong Kong Noodle Co. (2350), which is as unadorned as the vast range of noodles made fresh there daily.

- When you reach W. 24th Pl., turn west, go halfway down the block, and stop at tiny Sun Yat Sen Park. Hard by the maze of expressway on-ramps, the old men who play Chinese checkers here are unfazed by the racket.

- Now reverse course to Wentworth, walk north to W. 23rd St. and turn west. Mid-block on the north side, look for an otherwise unremarkable four-story brick structure looming over its neighbors. Now home to the Chinese-American Museum of Chicago, it has had a life that mirrored the community since its birth in 1896 (note the date near the roof); most recently it was a tofu factory. The museum is just getting off the ground, but the Chinese community is providing lavish funding.

- Continue to the end of the block, turn north on S. Princeton Ave. and then almost immediately turn east on one of Chicago's shortest named streets, W. Alexander St. Halfway down its 700-foot length, look for St. Therese Catholic Church. Built in 1904 to serve the Italians that lived here, it has now taken on Chinese trappings, right down to the lions out front. It manages to touch many bases in immigrant-heavy Chicago: masses are said in Cantonese, Mandarin, Indonesian and Italian. Inside there are numerous Chinese details such as decorative bamboo, and one holdover from the Italian era: the large crucifixion statue to the left of the altar was donated by Al Capone's mother.

- Return to Wentworth and walk north, crossing S. Cermak Rd. and turning southwest. If you think the firehouse at 212 is picture perfect, you're in agreement with Ron Howard, who used it as the main station for the firefighters in *Backdraft*.

- At the corner, cross S. Archer Ave. and walk down S. Princeton Ave. for barely 150 feet. Turn into the central passage of the Chinatown Square commercial development. For years Chinatown was hopelessly hemmed in by expressways and railroads. North of Archer, the old Santa Fe Railroad had a huge yard for trains like the legendary Super Chief. When these tracks were abandoned in the 1970s, development became possible, from the huge residential neighborhoods of the South Loop to Chinatown's expansion. As you walk amidst the shops, you'll see a cross-section of every kind of business you might find in Hong Kong or Beijing. Worth a sniff is Yin Wall, a ginseng emporium at 2112A.

Chinatown

● In the middle of Chinatown Square, a large public square has a variety of displays and sculptures, some informative and some hopelessly treacly. Look for the plaques touting Chinese inventions such as printing, paper-making, gunpowder, the compass and more. Among the statues of the zodiac signs is an especially winsome rabbit.

● Exit the northeast end of Chinatown Square and follow S. Wells St. through oodles of uninspired new housing blocks for about 200 yards to the stub end of W. 19th St. and turn west, crossing under the El and over some tracks to Ping Tom Park. You can't help but sigh as you reach this 12-acre oasis in the midst of the city. Opened in 1999, it is named for a long-time Chinatown leader who negotiated the development of the old rail yards. Stroll the paths, noting details like the bamboo patches and gingko trees. This may well be the place where the oft-maligned South Branch of the Chicago River is at its best. Look south to the massive lift bridge over the river. At 195 feet, the twin towers are the very embodiment of Chicago's industrial might in the early 20th century. Today Amtrak trains cross where once-famous names like the Broadway Limited passed years earlier.

● Return to W. 19th St., walk east and turn south on S. Wentworth Ave. Walk three blocks south until you reach Cermak. On the northwest corner, Three Happiness is popular for its lunchtime dim sum, with wheeled carts bearing treats circulating continuously.

● Walk east on Cermak, stopping at the Nine Dragon Wall, which boasts a fire-breathing 3,000 glazed tiles along its 36-foot-long length.

● End your walk at the Red Line El Cermak-Chinatown stop.

CONNECTING THE WALKS

At the end of this walk, you can link up with Walk 13 from the South Loop.

POINTS OF INTEREST

Won Kow 2237 S. Wentworth Ave., 312-842-7500

Emperor's Choice 2238 S. Wentworth Ave., 312-225-8800

Sun Sun Tong 2260 S. Wentworth Ave., 312-842-6398

Ten Ren Tea and Ginseng 2247 S. Wentworth Ave., 312-842-1171

Hong Kong Noodle Co. 2350 S. Wentworth Ave., 312-842-0480

Chiu Quon Bakery and Cafe 2242 S. Wentworth Ave., 312-225-6608

Chinese-American Museum of Chicago 238 W. 23rd St., 312-949-1000

Yin Wall 2112A S. Archer Ave., 312-225-2888

Three Happiness 209 W. Cermak Rd., 312-842-1964

route summary

1. Start facing the Chinese Gate over S. Wentworth Ave.
2. Walk south on Wentworth.
3. When you reach W. 24th Pl., turn right, go halfway down the block and stop at tiny Sun Yat Sen Park.
4. Return to Wentworth, walk north to W. 23rd St. and turn left.
5. Turn right on S. Princeton Ave. and then almost immediately turn right on W. Alexander St.
6. Return to Wentworth and turn left, crossing S. Cermak Rd. and turning southwest.
7. At the corner, cross S. Archer Ave. and walk down S. Princeton Ave. for barely 150 feet. Turn into the central passage of the Chinatown Square commercial development.
8. Exit the northeast end of Chinatown Square and follow S. Wells St. for about 200 yards to the stub end of W. 19th St. and turn left, crossing under the El and over some tracks to Ping Tom Park.
9. Return to W. 19th St. and turn right on S. Wentworth Ave. Walk three blocks until you reach Cermak.
10. Turn left and walk east on Cermak.
11. End your walk at the Red Line El Cermak-Chinatown stop.

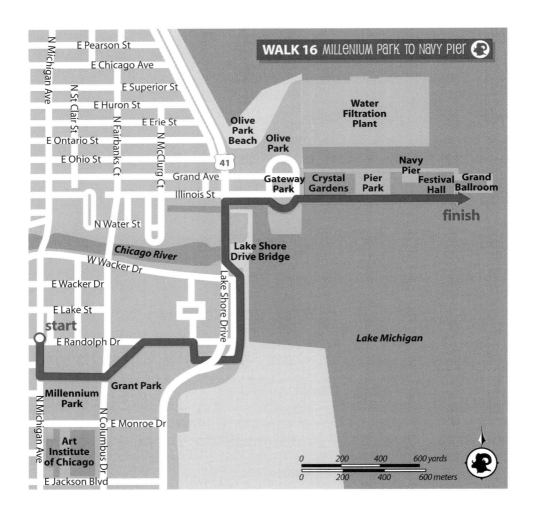

N Michigan Ave
E Pearson St
E Chicago Ave
N St Clair St
E Superior St
N Fairbanks Ct
E Huron St
E Erie St
N McClurg Ct
E Ontario St
E Ohio St
Grand Ave
Illinois St
41
Olive Park Beach
Olive Park
Gateway Park
Crystal Gardens
Pier Park
Navy Pier
Festival Hall
Grand Ballroom
Water Filtration Plant
finish

N Water St
Chicago River
W Wacker Dr
E Wacker Dr
Lake Shore Drive Bridge
E Lake St
Lake Shore Drive
start
E Randolph Dr
Grant Park
Lake Michigan

N Michigan Ave
N Columbus Dr
Millennium Park
E Monroe Dr
Art Institute of Chicago
E Jackson Blvd

0 200 400 600 yards
0 200 400 600 meters

16 MILLENNIUM PARK TO NAVY PIER: THINK BIG

BOUNDARIES: E. Grand Ave., Lake Michigan, E. Monroe St., N. Michigan Ave.
DISTANCE: 2½ miles
PUBLIC TRANSIT: Multiple bus and El lines serving the Loop

Just imagine if Daniel Burnham, instead of saying "Make no little plans. They have no magic to stir men's blood and probably will not themselves be realized," had said: "Make little plans, they'll keep your blood pressure low and come in on budget." Then Chicago would look like Schaumburg. This walk shows the Burnham ethos in action—for better or worse. From the grand spectacle that is Millennium Park, past Chicago's largest development, around a reversed river, past what might become the world's tallest condos, and on to Chicago's oddest amusement park, Navy Pier, is a walk of extremes, so take no little steps.

● Start your walk at the southeast corner of E. Randolph St. and N. Michigan Ave. Before you lies Millennium Park, Chicago's crowd-pleasing spectacle of public space. Most people know that the park's superlatives include the truly once-in-a-millennium blown budget (final cost $500 million, three times over) and blown timetable (opened in 2004, four years late for the timetable and name). But few care, as there's enough here to please even the grimmest curmudgeon (and a read of the budget might just make them happy in a Scrooge-ish kind of way). One thing to note: as costs spiraled, it was decided by the project's backers (a Who's Who of moneyed folks needing something to chat about at the club) to sell the naming rights to pretty much everything. In the narrative that follows, each brand name is lettered. Some are correct, others are made up for features that don't—yet—sport branding. Answers at the end.

● Promenade south through the ordered shrubbery of the Wrigley (a) Square Monument along Michigan Ave. The Viagra (b) Fountain spurts regularly. Soon you'll encounter the McCormick Tribune (c) Plaza and Ice Rink. It's a great spot to watch the Tonya Hardings of tomorrow all winter long.

● Continue south along Michigan to the Crown (d) Fountain. One of the most popular parts of the park, two 50-foot monoliths face each other across a reflecting pool. And when we say face, we mean face. The glass blocks are one huge video installation showing the faces of Chicagoans. Every so often one of them puckers their lips and the Gatorade (e) stream of water shoots out, dousing all nearby. On hot days, it's a mesmerizing and way-cool delight.

- Ascend the Roto-Rooter (f) stairs toward the rear of Crown Fountain and follow the crowds slightly north to the Chase (g) Promenade Central and the Charmin (h) *Cloud Gate,* which is far more commonly called "The Bean." This mirrored legume is truly a hoot and watching the reflections of others and the clouds above is a nice way to waste some time.

- Head east via the jobs.com (i) promenade to the walkway surrounding the Ortho (j) Great Lawn, which is the home to open-air concerts all summer long. At the north end, you won't miss the stunning metallic explosion that is the Jay Pritzker (k) Pavilion. Most agree that the Frank Gehry-designed work is worth its over-budget figure of 558 percent.

- Follow the walkway south to the Laurie (l) Garden, home of the *Chicago Sun-Times* (m) shrub and the *Playboy* (n) bush. It's worth picking up a guide or joining a tour, as pretty much every plant here relates to Chicago. Note that the Colgate (o) Bridge shooting south of here will link the park to the vast new addition to the Art Institute.

- Stroll northwest and take the BP (p) Bridge over N. Columbus Dr. This Gehry-designed sinuous dream of a path has drawn some criticism as being a "bridge to nowhere," since at the east end the attractions are much more rooted in the ground and only carry the branding "Chicago Park District."

- The portion of Grant Park north of E. Monroe St. has always been something of a forgotten step-child. But lately it's been much in the spotlight. There's the bridge from Millennium Park, huge new development just north (more on this in a moment), and a very controversial proposal to bring the Chicago Children's Museum here from Navy Pier. We'll leave the fulminations to others (the tenor is like locking Bill O'Reilly in a room with Keith Olbermann), and instead suggest you make your way through the complex geometry of the plantings in a northeasterly direction until you are on the top level of E. Randolph St.

- Stop where N. Field Blvd. intersects with Randolph and look north. This is the heart of Lakeshore East. You'll see the attempt to finally finish the enormous Illinois Center project begun in the 1960s. (See sidebar "What Lies Below" on p. 125.) Amidst the smattering of high-rises built over the last 40 years (and whose unifying design element is "ugly"), are seven new ones, out of a planned 18. Some will reach over 80 stories. Already complete is a 6-acre park in the middle that has hopefully been planted with shade-tolerant grass, as the ring of surrounding towers is going to be a major sun-block. It's a vast $4 billion investment—and that's if the Millennium Park folks don't get hold of the budget.

- Cross Randolph and return to Grant Park. Follow the paths east through the rather restfully unadorned trapezoid of trees and grass between Lake Shore Dr. and Randolph. Cross under LSD and emerge at the waterfront.

- Ahead of you is DuSable Harbor. To the right, that old tub is the home of the Columbia Yacht Club, a refreshingly unstuffy operation. On Wednesday nights in season, it holds regattas called Beer Cans, with the express purpose of having fun. Many members have their boats moored here. As you walk along, you may try to look your best in order to score an invite aboard for a gin and tonic (note that people of a certain gender, age, and hair color seem to do best at this).

- Walk north along the water until you reach the acronym-laden monument of the American Society of Civil Engineers (ASCE), which honors what is essentially the bowl of your toilet. To explain: until the 1880s, Chicago's wastewater went into Lake Michigan, where it tended to foul

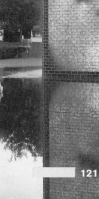

Crown Fountain, Millennium Park

the brackish waters of the swampy shoreline and the city's source of water; cholera was just one problem. Then city engineers hit upon a brilliant scheme: reverse the flow of the Chicago River. Vast canals were built and the river indeed did then flow south. One resident 60 miles downstream wondered why Chicago had the right to send "sickness and death" his way. No matter, Chicago had the clout and locals were far happier knowing that what they flushed away would eventually flow past New Orleans, as opposed to out their faucets. The long low structures to the east are the locks that ensure the Chicago River directly to the north always keeps flowing the wrong way.

- Walk west and ascend the path to the lower level of the Lake Shore Dr. Bridge. Cross north and stop once you're over dry land. This is not the handiest vantage point, but to your immediate west is the site of the Chicago Spire, the 2000-square-foot, 150-story residential tower that's meant to be the tallest structure in North America (Dubai and Asia have locks on even taller buildings). Depending on the economy and sales of the multi-million-dollar condos, it may be done by 2011. The architect, Calatrava, says the soaring, narrow and complex spiral shape is inspired by nature; he probably doesn't mean the rather similar spirochetes that cause Lyme disease or syphilis.

- Still on the bridge, look east at the nub of land jutting into the water. For over 20 years, this well-located but derelict plot of land has been designated as the future home of DuSable Park. Lack of funding and will have held things up, but now it may become parkland yet as part of the Chicago Spire project. One hitch: you may notice a certain glow at night. The soil may be radioactive from this area's industrial days, when it was home to a manufacturer of luminescent dials.

- Take the stairs down to the landscaped area just south of E. Illinois St. below the bridge. Walk east until you reach the promenade along the south side of Navy Pier.

- Built in 1916, Navy Pier handled freight throughout World War II. Later it was used as the first campus of the University of Illinois at Chicago, and then for not much at all. In 1995 it received a zillion-dollar reconstruction (in pre-Millennium Park dollars) that turned it into part fun fest, part exhibition space. As you walk east along its more

BACK STORY: WHAT LIES BELOW

Millennium Park and Grant Park were once Lake Michigan. After the fire in 1871, rubble was used to build up land toward the shore we see today. The Chicago Cubs even had a diamond here pre-1900, when for a time they a) didn't suck, and b) were known as the Orphans. The Illinois Central Railroad had vast rail yards north of E. Monroe St. throughout World War II, and a station at Randolph St. that's still used by Metra and has been renamed Millennium Station. The area north of E. Randolph St. became known as Illinois Center in the 1960s, and various bits of land under the triple-deck roads have been parking lots, a golf course and the auto pound for towed cars.

than half-mile-long promenade, the pier is broken into various zones that mix the high-brow (theaters etc.) with the low-brow (franchised restaurants like the tired Bubba Gump's), and might even cause you to raise an eyebrow. A few highlights heading east: until it relocates someplace, the Chicago Children's Museum; the Crystal Gardens, a genuinely delightful spot, especially on a rainy day; the Carousel— if you can get past the McDonald's branding; Chicago Shakespeare Theater, which specializes in the works of Franz Liebkind, er, no; and WBEZ, Chicago's NPR station and home to shows like *This American Life*. At the very end, the Grand Ballroom is a grand space. There's a summertime beer garden here, and views from the tip back to the ever-growing Chicago skyline.

● From Navy Pier, you can catch the 29 State and 65 Grand busses west to the Red Line El stop at Grand.

Answers: The following brands are not sponsors of attractions in Millennium Park– yet: b, e, f, h, i, j, m, n, o

POINTS OF INTEREST

Navy Pier www.navypier.com, 312-595-7437

Chicago Children's Museum 312-527-1000

Chicago Shakespeare Theater www.chicagoshakes.com, 312-595-5600

ROUTE SUMMARY

1. Start at the southeast corner of E. Randolph St. and N. Michigan Ave.

2. Walk south along Michigan Ave. to the Crown Fountain.

3. Ascend the stairs toward the rear of Crown Fountain and go slightly north to the Chase Promenade Central.

4. Head east via the promenade to the walkway surrounding Great Lawn.

5. Follow the walkway south to the Laurie Garden.

6. Stroll northwest and take the BP Bridge over N. Columbus Dr.

7. Walk in a northeasterly direction until you are on the top level of E. Randolph St.

8. Stop where N. Field Blvd. intersects with Randolph.

9. Re-cross Randolph and return to Grant Park. Follow the paths east through the green area between Lake Shore Dr. and Randolph. Cross under LSD and emerge at the waterfront.

10. Walk north along the water.

11. Walk west and ascend the path to the lower level of the Lake Shore Dr. Bridge.

12. Take the stairs down to the landscaped area just south of E. Illinois St. below the bridge. Walk east until you reach the promenade along the south side of Navy Pier.

13. Walk to the east end of the pier.

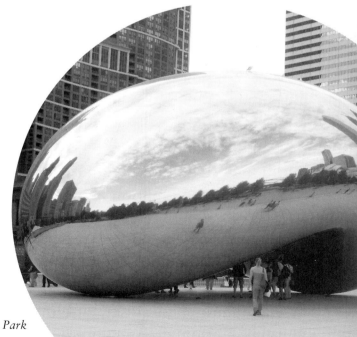

Cloud Gate *(a.k.a. "The Bean"), Millennium Park*

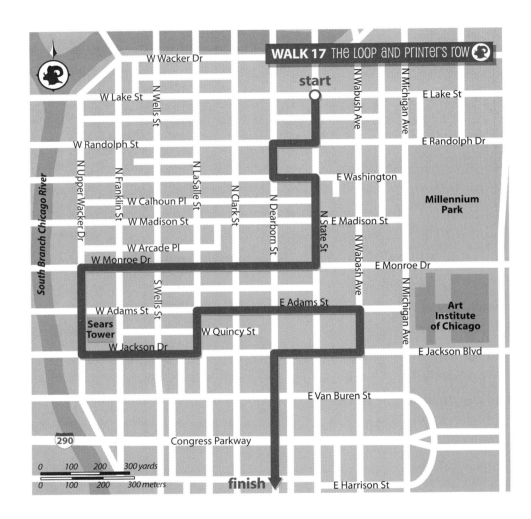

start

W Wacker Dr

W Lake St

N Wells St

E Lake St

N Wabush Ave

N Michigan Ave

E Randolph Dr

W Randolph St

E Washington

Millennium
Park

N Upper Wacker Dr

N Franklin St

W Calhoun Pl

N LaSalle St

N Clark St

N Dearborn St

N State St

E Madison St

South Branch Chicago River

W Madison St

W Arcade Pl

W Monroe Dr

E Monroe Dr

N Wabash Ave

N Michigan Ave

Art
Institute
of Chicago

W Adams St

S Wells St

E Adams St

Sears
Tower

W Quincy St

E Jackson Blvd

W Jackson Dr

E Van Buren St

290

Congress Parkway

0   100   200   300 yards

0   100   200   300 meters

finish

E Harrison St

17 THE LOOP AND PRINTER'S ROW: LANDMARKS NEW AND OLD

BOUNDARIES: **Lake St., Wabash St., Polk St., S. Wacker Dr.**
DISTANCE: **2½ miles**
PUBLIC TRANSIT: **All El lines converge on the Loop.**

Tour groups crisscross the Loop in any weather and with good reason: it's home to an astonishing array of architecture spanning 150 years. Tens of thousands more people cram its canyons on weekdays for work, while at night crowds enjoy its many theaters. Some even stick around to slumber the night away in one of the multiplying number of condos. This walk through the Loop and the Printer's Row district just south covers landmarks both famous and not-so-famous. Even for such a familiar place, it still has its surprises.

- **Start your tour under the decrepit Lake St. El station above the intersection of Lake St. and N. State St. Beloved only by pigeons (look out!) and transit geeks, this hulk of a station dates back to 1895 when the "Loop" of track around downtown was built, providing both transport and a handy nickname for the district.**

- **Walk south on State St. The block between Lake St. and Randolph St. is ripe with entertainment. Immediately on your right is ABC7 (a.k.a. WLS-TV). Note the ground floor studios so that you can watch anchors reading the newscasts. Also note that reflective barriers inside will prevent them from being distracted by your idiotic gestures outside.**

- **On the east side of the block, the Chicago Theater embodies one of the great surviving marquees from the era of grand movie palaces. Back on the west side, look for the small entrance to the Gene Siskel Film Center. Named for the late, famed film reviewer, the center is part of the Film Center of the School of the Art Institute and shows the kind of off-beat and unusual films you won't find on airplanes or on the sale racks at Wal-Mart. Off the lobby upstairs, there's a now bittersweet Skrebneski portrait of Siskel and his TV-partner Roger Ebert when both were in their prime.**

- At the intersection with Randolph St., you won't miss the jiffy new Joffrey Tower on the northeast corner. Named for the dance company, which occupies two of the lower floors, it is yet another condo tower. Twenty years ago the residential population of the Loop was a few hundred; now, with new buildings like the Joffrey and conversions of older ones with floors sizes too small for business, the population is in the thousands and growing with the opening of every new project. Where the condo portion of the building is set back from the lower level, there's a "green roof," a plant-heavy space meant to be more environmentally friendly. After Mayor Daley said he liked them, politically savvy developers started installing them all over town.

- Walk west on Randolph. To your left is the vast new development officially—and dully—dubbed 108 N. State St. During the decades when it was derelict, this prime bit of Loop real estate was known as Block 37. The list of failed developments here reads like a list of Bush Administration plans for Iraq. The complex you see now includes the requisite "upscale" mall, condos and a new CTA station to serve the Blue Line under Dearborn St. and the Red Line under State St.

- At N. Dearborn St., pause and take in the comparatively small Delaware Building on the northeast corner. It was built shortly after the 1871 fire and is one of very few this old left in the Loop.

- Walk south on Dearborn, noting the iconic Picasso sculpture in Daley Plaza. Try to decide what it is—Pablo never said, although it resembles both his wife and dog at the time he designed it in 1965 (obviously his dog was very attractive . . .).

- Turn east on W. Washington St. This corner of the 108 N. State St. building is where CBS2 (a.k.a. WBBM-TV) has its studios. You can moon all you want, but nobody (other than your mother, someplace) will notice.

- Stop at the intersection with N. State St. Few welcomed the arrival of Macy's when it subsumed locally beloved Marshall Field's, and it's been a rocky relationship since. One hopes this huge and grand store hangs on as part of a vast chain. One positive: chef Rick Bayless has opened a "quick-serve" (as opposed to fast-food) version of his always jammed Frontera Grill in River North. On the northeast corner, ponder the exquisite gleaming terra-cotta façade on the Reliance Building (a.k.a. Hotel Burnham). That this 1890s masterpiece was decades ahead of its time is a given.

- Walk south on State St., the "great street" that has been given new life thanks to every discount chain that ever graced a suburban strip mall. Stop at the intersection with Madison St., ground zero for Chicago's surprisingly brilliant street numbering system. On the southeast corner is the Sullivan Center, the all-but-unknown new name for the Carson, Pirie, Scott and Company building here. The façade, especially the iron grillwork at the corner, is a work of art by Louis Sullivan dating to 1899. Unlike Field's, the departure of Carson's was not mourned; their merchandising had been strictly Bulgarian for some time.

- Turn west on W. Monroe St. At the intersection with S. Dearborn St., look to the northwest corner for a bit of public art that's rare because people actually like it: Marc Chagall's *Four Seasons*. The complex's name this week is Chase Plaza, although it's just another couple of mergers away from Mega-Monopoly Plaza.

- Walking west, stop at S. LaSalle St. to take in the famous canyon of the financial and legal district. Look up to see the statue of Ceres, Roman goddess of agriculture, atop the 45-story Art Deco Chicago Board of Trade Building.

- Stay with the setting sun (it's there behind the many towers) and walk to the intersection with S. Wacker Dr. Several striking high-rises have been built here of late, including the elliptical sweep of the Hyatt Center (2005) on the northeast corner. The stainless steel and aquamarine glass here catch reflections all day long.

- Walk south on Wacker until you are hard by the ebony shaft of the Sears Tower. The tallest building in the world when it opened in 1971, the 110 stories here still pack a

Board of Trade Building and LaSalle St.

vertical punch. On the W. Jackson Blvd. side, pause at the entrance to the Skydeck on the 103rd floor. On the plus side: on clear days, unparalleled views of the city and four states. On the minus side: insipid introduction movie, public spaces that would have been cutting edge at the 1980 Moscow Olympics, hour-long waits in summer and often-filthy windows. We prefer the Hancock (see Walk 20).

- Head east. Just past S. LaSalle St., look for the little plaza just east of the Board of Trade building. Two stern statues on plinths here have stories almost as dramatic as their expressions: key elements of the previous Board of Trade building, they ended up lost in suburban landfill (!) after it was demolished in 1929. Rediscovered, they can be enjoyed again today.

- Walk north on LaSalle St. to W. Adams St. The entire southeast portion of the block is taken up with the iconic Rookery Building, an 1885 Burnham and Root masterpiece. Like a perfectly ripe apple, the outside is pretty enough, but plunge inside for the real reward, in this case the astonishing sky-lit lobby.

- Go east on Adams. As you cross S. Dearborn St., spare a nod to Alexander Calder's *Flamingo* on its Federal Plaza perch (and if it's Tuesday and temperate, check out one of the city's best farmers markets).

- Midblock on W. Adams St. after Dearborn, you'll see the stylish and timeless sign for the beloved Berghoff restaurant and bar. But save your warm thoughts for the sign, as all is not well inside. In a prime example of why business owners should protect their legacies, a Berghoff granddaughter took over the place in 2006 and rather ludicrously renamed it "17/West at the Berghoff." Gone is much of the classic menu, the veteran—and unionized—employees, and the crowds. When we stopped by on a Friday afternoon, the bar that would have once been packed with everyone from judges to teamsters was virtually empty.

- Continue across State St. until you reach S. Wabash St., and turn south. Stroll this block very slowly, not for any one highlight but rather just to soak up a classic slice of the Loop: the mix of vintage buildings, scruffy businesses and most importantly, the road of the El overhead.

- Turn west on E. Jackson Blvd. and walk slowly. Just before you reach the rather tasty Fontano's Subs, look for the minute alley on your right. Once a private drive called Pickwick Alley, the structure deep in its shadows at the back likely dates back to at least 1857, making it the oldest—and most forgotten—building in the Loop.

- As you cross State St. heading west, your nose may hijack your route right into the Garrett Popcorn shop on the northwest corner. Trust us, the caramel and cheese corns are simply divine—and calorie-free on any day ending in "y."

- At S. Dearborn St. turn south, walk slowly and crane your neck. On your right is the landmark Monadnock Building, once briefly in 1889 the tallest building in the world. It was also one of the last tall structures to be built out of brick; just note the massive lower walls, with windows punched through, that look like battlements. Now look left as you pass midblock and behold the Fisher Building. Built only seven years later (1896), it, like the Reliance Building, had an interior steel frame that allowed glass-covered walls that need only support their own weight. Note the plethora of fishy details on the riotous terra-cotta façade. A lavish restoration in 2001 made the inside worth a visit.

- Stop when you reach W. Congress Pkwy. and look back north from the northwest corner. You can appreciate the often overlooked Manhattan Building (1891) at 431, the Plymouth Building (1899) at 417, and the Old Colony Building (1894) at 407. Line up the last one with the Fisher Building, and you'll note how one or both has relaxed its posture in old age.

- South of Congress, Dearborn is the spine of Printer's Row, so named for the scores of printers that operated here from the 1880s to the 1950s. They left behind dozens of beautiful buildings that today have been rehabbed into loft apartments. It's a pleasant neighborhood, which writes a new chapter for itself every June during the annual book fair.

- A few highlights: The 1911 Transportation Building (600), at the southwest corner with W. Harrison St., was where Eliot Ness had his office during the peak "Untouchables" years in the 1930s; Kasey's Tavern (701) has a battered, curved wooden bar from 1889; and Sandmeyer's Bookstore (714), is a fine indie that does well by the local history.

- Pause for a couple moments by the tiny fountain on Printer's Square just north of Sandmeyer's. The vast hulk of the 1909 building to the west on S. Federal St. replaced dozens of buildings from an era when hardback and binding meant something else in the neighborhood. A rather delightful 1896 screed on the immorality of Chicago titled *If Christ Came to Chicago* shows that on this block alone there were 35 brothels.

- Finish your walk where Dearborn dead-ends into W. Polk St. The soaring brick clock tower marks Dearborn Station, where famous Santa Fe Railroad trains like the Super Chief (40 hours to Los Angeles) once arrived and departed. It's now the front for vast residential developments that stretch south for almost 2 miles.

- Head over to S. State St. to the Red Line El stop at Harrison.

CONNECTING THE WALKS

At the end of the walk, go south four blocks and join Walks 13 and 23.

POINTS OF INTEREST

Gene Siskel Film Center 164 N. State St., 312-846-2800

Frontera Fresco Macy's, 111 N. State St., 312-781-4483

Sears Tower Skydeck 233 S. Wacker Dr., 312-875-9447

17/West at the Berghoff 17 W. Adams St., 312-427-3170

Fontano's Subs 20 E. Jackson Blvd., 312-663-3061

Garrett Popcorn 2 W. Jackson Blvd., 312-360-1108

Kasey's Tavern 701 S. Dearborn St., 312-427-7992

Sandmeyer's Bookstore 714 S. Dearborn St., 312-922-2104

route summary

1. Start at the Lake St. El station above the intersection of Lake St. and N. State St.
2. Walk south on State St.
3. Turn right on Randolph.
4. Turn left on N. Dearborn Ave.
5. Turn left on W. Washington St.
6. Turn right and walk south on State St.
7. Turn right on W. Monroe St.
8. Turn left and walk south on S. Wacker Dr.
9. Turn left on W. Jackson Blvd.
10. Turn left on LaSalle St. and walk north to W. Adams St.
11. Go right on Adams.
12. Turn right on S. Wabash St.
13. Turn right on E. Jackson Blvd.
14. At S. Dearborn St. turn left.
15. Finish your walk where Dearborn dead-ends into W. Polk St.

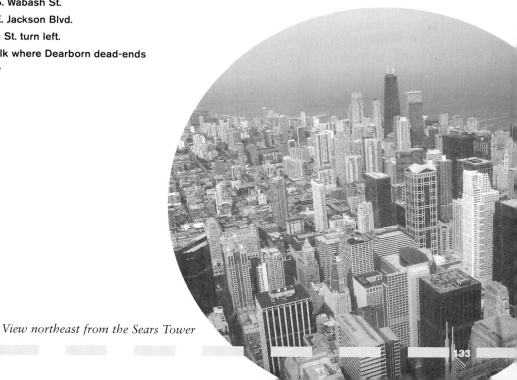

View northeast from the Sears Tower

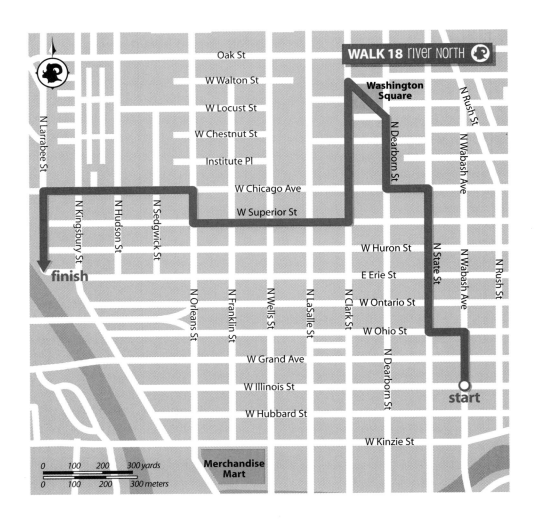

Washington
Square

Oak St

W Walton St

W Locust St

W Chestnut St

Institute Pl

W Chicago Ave

W Superior St

W Huron St

E Erie St

W Ontario St

W Ohio St

W Grand Ave

W Illinois St

W Hubbard St

W Kinzie St

N Larrabee St

N Kingsbury St

N Hudson St

N Sedgwick St

N Orleans St

N Franklin St

N Wells St

N LaSalle St

N Clark St

N Dearborn St

N Dearborn St

N State St

N Wabash Ave

N Wabash Ave

N Rush St

N Rush St

finish

start

Merchandise
Mart

0   100   200   300 yards

0   100   200   300 meters

18 rIVer NOrTH: Break THe SHackLes anD escape THe CHains

BOUNDARIES: W. Walton St., N. Wabash Ave., Illinois St., North Branch of the Chicago River
DISTANCE: 1¾ miles
PUBLIC TRANSIT: Numerous bus lines and the Red Line El to Grand

Once the marshy home to Chicago's earliest non-indigenous citizens, who needed a place to rest between explorations, River North is now where non-locals need a rest after a night of urban frolic. The blocks east of N. Dearborn St. heave at night with funseekers, finding all they could hope for in huge venues, many of which are chains. Amidst all this, the ceaseless addition of condo and apartment towers boosts the permanent population prowling the sidewalks. To the west, River North is given over to a plethora of galleries and loft-conversions.

● Start your walk at the point on N. Wabash Ave. where it passes over E. Illinois St. To the southeast, the otherwise unremarkable old building housing the Jazz Record Mart (probably the best of its kind in the world!) sits about on the spot where John Kinzie, Chicago's first white settler, had his house. A fur trader, Kinzie lived in the cabin that had first been built here by Jean Baptiste Point DuSable, Chicago's first non-Indian resident (he hailed from the Caribbean). Typical of the rough-edged frontier folk of the time, Kinzie set the tone for the city by doing whatever it took to get ahead. In 1812 he kept selling rot-gut booze to the Indians right up until the Fort Dearborn massacre (see Walk 13). The same year he claimed "self-defense" in the killing of a business rival, whose remains were found during excavations for the building in front of you in 1891.

● Walk down and north on Wabash, crossing E. Grand Ave. Do your best to avert your eyes from the P. F. Changs on the northwest corner, lest you turn into a pillar of salt. This part of River North, just west of N. Michigan Ave., is wildly popular with suburbanites, who flock to chain restaurants like Chang's that are identical to ones at strip malls near their homes. Go figure. Also, a) we're not going to tell you where to find the Red Lobster, and b) we won't mention what happened to *South Park*'s Randy Marsh when he ate at Chang's.

- At E. Ohio St., turn west. You'll note the lines at the southwest corner for Pizzeria Uno. This is really the place where Ike Sewell claimed to have invented Chicago-style deep dish pizza in 1943. Note two things: 1) the originals here and a block away at Pizzeria Due are much better than their franchised variations, and 2) several others claimed to have invented Chicago-style pizza, and many years ago the vitriol around the claims assumed almost Kinzie-esque proportions.

- Turn north on N. State St. and pause to admire the Tree Studios, an 1894 creation that was designed to entice artists to live in Chicago. Above the ground-floor shops were studio apartments with huge west-facing windows. This arrangement lasted through the 1990s, but the area's rampant commercialization caught up with the building in 2004 when the last of the artists were booted and rows of upscale boutiques installed. Shed a tear for Pops for Champagne on the Ohio corner. This once-heavenly Lincoln Park gem moved here, and now cleans up selling small pours of expensive champagne to mobs for whom Miller is really the champagne of beers.

- At the corner of Erie St. and N. State St., Bijan's Bistro is definitely the only place in town you can chow down first on escargot followed by steak au poivre after 2 AM. Long a River North stalwart in various iterations, Bijan's is heaven for night owls who need to nail a snail. (The wine list is good too.)

- Continue north on State St. to Superior St. Given the range of drop-dead (so to speak) gorgeous churches in Chicago, Holy Name Cathedral on the northeast corner is surprisingly modest. Still, it has solid details and you feel a certain majesty inside, knowing you are in the primo church of one of the largest Roman Catholic dioceses in the world. If you also feel a little hint of hell, just go across State St. to the parking lot, scene of two of Chicago's most notorious gangland hits of the Roaring 20s. Clichés come from somewhere, and the Chicago mobs supplied all of them: In 1924, North Side boss Dion O'Banion was trimming posies in his flower shop at 738 N. State when several men thought to be in the employ of Al Capone walked in and shot him. Two years later, O'Banion's successor and virulent Capone-rival Earl "Hymie" Weiss was crossing State St. toward the flower shop when five Tommy guns opened up from an apartment at 740 N. State. Death was immediate. (And only after tourists had gawked for years did the archdiocese finally fix the substantial bullet damage to the front of the cathedral.)

- Walk west one block on W. Chicago Ave. and turn north on N. Dearborn St. Given that high-rise apartments/condos have been exploding out of the ground in River North like tulips in the spring, that there are some original residences in the next two blocks is remarkable. The row houses at 802-812 and 827-833 date from the 1870s and provide a contrast between elegant European and classic Chicago brick.

- At Delaware Pl. take a stroll into Washington Square Park, a now-peaceful place with a colorful past. In the 1920s and 1930s it was known as "Bughouse Square" because it was the center of Chicago's robust free-speech movement. On many days crowds would gather to hear speakers discourse on subjects as diverse as communism, free love, the high price of gas, and more. Look for a plaque commemorating this at the west end. In 1970 it was the center of the city's first Gay Pride March. On the north side, the grand lines of the 1890 Newberry Library (a private research facility open to the public) provide a mannered backdrop.

- Exit the park and walk south on N. Clark St., crossing W. Chicago Ave. Let the vintage STOP & DRINK sign be your beacon into the Clark St. Ale House, a long-running local with a superb collection of Midwestern microbrews. (Previously the bar was called the Stop & Drink. It was known for its lack of windows, cheap lager and continuous porn on the TVs.) If you hear gunshots, they're probably coming from the oft-shuttered nightclub just south, where several Chicago Bears have come to headline-grabbing grief.

- Follow the siren song of another classic Chicago tavern by walking west two blocks from Clark St. on W. Superior St. to the northeast corner with N. Wells St. The Brehon

Erie Street Park

137

Pub dates from the 1800s and is little changed. Among its keg-full of stories: in 1978 the *Chicago Sun-Times* at its journalistic peak bought the place, named it "The Mirage" and staffed the bar with reporters. A "Mr. Fix-it" soon arrived and guided them through the process of bribing all manner of city inspectors and other officials. However, he drew the line at the Chicago Police, saying: "if you pay off a cop, they keep coming around every month, like flies, looking for a payoff." The resulting stories ran for 25 days. (Two of the reporters wrote a delightful book on the escapade—*The Mirage: A Tale of Cold Beer and Hot Graft,* from Marion Street Press, 2008.)

● Suitably fortified, walk west. You're in the heart of one of Chicago's main gallery districts. There are literally dozens in the blocks around the intersection of Superior and N. Franklin St. (under the El). Just a couple of recommendations: the 300 W. Superior building is filled with galleries, including the Judy Saslow Gallery, which has a carefully chosen selection of local artists entering their prime; and the building at 311, which includes the Stephen Daiter Gallery, known for its shows of photographers such as Chicago treasure Art Shay.

● Walk one block north on N. Orleans St. Turn west on Chicago Ave. In a small storefront on the south side (after, oh, four score and seven steps), look for the Abraham Lincoln Book Shop. Since 1938 it has cherished all things related to the 16th president, whose monumental legacy is honored by Illinois license plates ("Land of Lincoln") if not by the actions of its politicians. Among Lincoln's many quotes is his famous one on slavery: "A house divided against itself cannot stand."

● Continue west. As you pass N. Hudson Ave., look on the north side of the street for the fence bearing cheery signs that include GROW, PLAY and SHARE. This is the Chicago Avenue Community Garden, a venture of the Fourth Presbyterian Church (the ritzy Gothic number across from the John Hancock Center on N. Michigan Ave.) and the remaining residents of Cabrini-Green, the once-huge public housing projects that ran north all the way to North Ave. Their size was overshadowed only by their reputation, which was horrible. Now most of Cabrini—and the folks who lived there—are gone, replaced by developments that keep the minority poor in the minority. Those who remain can come here and plant something to see if it grows.

- Continuing west you reach one of the most ambitious reuse projects. The complex of buildings on and near the river was once home to Montgomery Ward, the little-missed department store chain that was forever in the shadow of Sears. The 1970s high-rise on the southeast corner of Chicago Ave. and N. Larrabee St. was the corporate headquarters. Now, where execs once anxiously awaited the overnight sales figures for polyester leisure suits and naugahyde sofas, upscale condo-dwellers cavort on satin sheets—or maybe they just watch their college team on ESPN. The ground floor is home to the posh Brasserie Ruhlmann, a pricey eatery named for the 1920s Parisian Art Deco designer. Run by the same locals behind trendy Japonais (in the old warehouse building on the northwest corner), the brasserie is doing everything to live down the reputation of its sibling in New York City, which got the sort of reviews often reserved for foamy fresh oysters. The stolid brick and concrete former warehouses on Larrabee face over 1,500 feet of the North Branch of the Chicago River. Look skyward for the wispy elegance of *Commerce*, the sprightly statue atop 619 W. Chicago.

- Head south on N. Larrabee St. to its end at W. Erie St. Ahead of you is Chicago's newest park, Erie Park, dedicated in 2006 and with a name that might as well be "The Name is Available to Honor Somebody Park." Although on the barren side now, the sloping, grassy site runs for over 350 scenic feet along the North Branch of the river and is a real breath of (sort of) fresh air. Find a shady spot under a young tree and absorb the city vista in front of you: architecture tour boats, cement barges, frazzled traffic zipping across the Ohio St. Bridge, commuter trains in the distance and O'Hare-bound planes overhead.

- To exit, walk three blocks north to catch a 66 Chicago bus or a half mile northeast to the Brown and Purple Lines El stop at Chicago.

POINTS OF INTErEST

Jazz Record Mart 27 E. Illinois St., 312-222-1467

Pizzeria Uno 29 E. Ohio St., 312-321-1000

Bijan's Bistro 633 N. State St., 312-202-1904

Newberry Library 60 W. Walton St., 312-255-3504

Clark St. Ale House 742 N. Clark St., 312-642-9253

Brehon Pub 731 N. Wells St., 312-642-1071

Judy Saslow Gallery 300 W. Superior St., 312-943-0530

Stephen Daiter Gallery 311 W. Superior St., 312-787-3350

Abraham Lincoln Book Shop 357 W. Chicago Ave., 312-944-3085

Brasserie Ruhlmann 500 W. Superior St., 312-494-1900

Japonais 600 W. Chicago Ave., 312-822-9600

rOUTE SUMMArY

1. Start at the point on N. Wabash Ave. where it passes over E. Illinois St.
2. Walk down and north on Wabash.
3. At E. Ohio St., turn left.
4. Turn right on N. State St.
5. Turn left and walk west one block on W. Chicago Ave., then turn right on N. Dearborn St.
6. At Delaware Pl. take a stroll into Washington Square Park.
7. Exit the park and walk south on N. Clark St.
8. Turn right on W. Superior St.
9. Turn right on N. Orleans St. and go north one block.
10. Turn left on W. Chicago Ave.
11. Turn left on N. Larrabee St. and walk south to its end at W. Erie St.

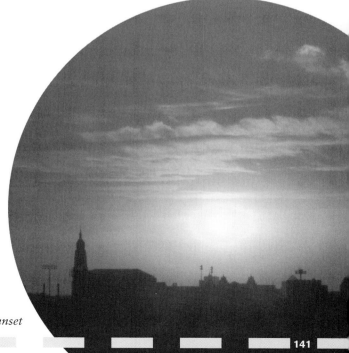

Chicago sunset

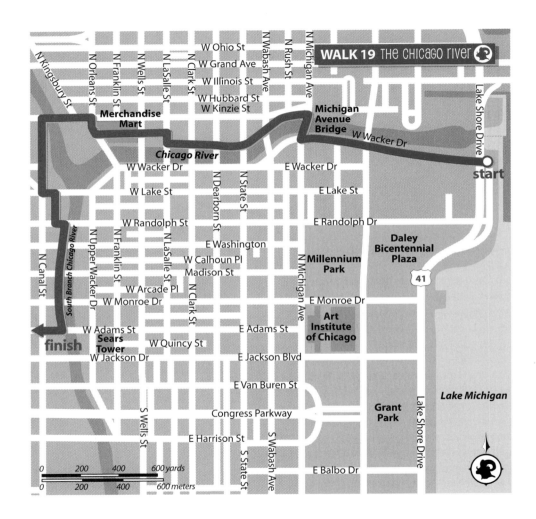

WALK 19 THE CHICAGO RIVER

N Kingsbury St
N Orleans St
N Franklin St
N Wells St
N LaSalle St
N Clark St
W Ohio St
W Grand Ave
W Illinois St
W Hubbard St
W Kinzie St
N Wabash Ave
N Rush St
N Michigan Ave

Merchandise Mart

Michigan Avenue Bridge
W Wacker Dr

Lake Shore Drive

Chicago River

W Wacker Dr
W Lake St
N Dearborn St
N State St
E Wacker Dr
E Lake St

start

W Randolph St
E Randolph Dr

Daley Bicentennial Plaza

N Canal St
South Branch Chicago River
N Upper Wacker Dr
N Franklin St
N LaSalle St
N Clark St
E Washington
W Calhoun Pl
Madison St
W Arcade Pl
W Monroe Dr
E Monroe Dr

Millennium Park
N Michigan Ave

Art Institute of Chicago

41

finish
Sears Tower
W Adams St
W Quincy St
W Jackson Dr
E Adams St
E Jackson Blvd

S Wells St
E Van Buren St

Congress Parkway
S State St
S Wabash Ave

E Harrison St

Grant Park

Lake Michigan

Lake Shore Drive

E Balbo Dr

0   200   400   600 yards
0   200   400   600 meters

19 THE CHICAGO RIVER: GO WITH THE FLOW

BOUNDARIES: **Chicago River, Lake Michigan, W. Adams St., Canal St.**
DISTANCE: **2½ miles**
PUBLIC TRANSIT: **6 Jackson Park Express bus to E. Wacker Dr. and then walk east, or 29 State, 65 Grand or 66 Chicago busses to Navy Pier and walk south over the river on lower Lake Shore Dr.**

First it was a lethargic little stream flowing into swamplands at Lake Michigan. Later it was a virtual downspout, wicking away Chicago's filth and corruption (well, some). For decades most people turned their backs on the river, only paying notice when barrels of green dye were dumped in on St. Patrick's Day. But in recent years, the Chicago River has gained much in reputation. From the industrial poetry of the bridges to the open vistas possible in the ever-more-crowded skyline, the river has come to be celebrated as the vital heart of downtown. The growing flotilla of tour boats and the lengthening strands of river walks allow ever-greater numbers of people to enjoy the river. This walk starts at the mouth of the Chicago River and follows it right to the far edge of the Loop

- Begin your walk at the mouth of the Chicago River, on the south bank just east of Lake Shore Dr. Take in the lock system that makes certain that the river—and what's in it—always flows away from the lake, and then point yourself downstream, i.e., west.

- It took until 2000 for a passage to be built that gives access to the river walk from the lake front but in this case it's much better late than never. The 170-foot-long tunnel under Lake Shore Dr. is lined with 16 murals by Ellen Lanyon that trace the human and natural history of the river.

- Emerging on the west side, walk along the grass and tree-lined river bank. You're down low so you can appreciate the boats that go by while the confection that is the Wrigley Building on the north side grows ever closer (also growing closer will be the enormous thing to the left of the Wrigley Building, on which more later). From down here you can see the ceaseless condo development in Streeterville, including the 2,000-foot-tall Chicago Spire near the mouth. What you can't see very well due to your proximity is the three-decked esthetic horror that Illinois Center shows to the river. As Lyndon Johnson said, sometimes it's better to be inside the tent.

- At the Michigan Ave. Bridge, climb 20 steps up to the hair-raising hell that is Lower Wacker Dr. Say your prayers and cross Lower Michigan Ave. to the base of the southwest tower of the bridge. Here you'll find the Bridgehouse and Chicago River Museum, a literally often-overlooked spot with surprisingly good displays, including the main one, which says it all: "Prairie stream, bustling port, city sewer, living treasure: the Chicago River."

- Climb to the upper level of the N. Michigan Ave. Bridge and cross north. Stop midway for a view that, particularly at sunset, may be one of Chicago's better "time to kiss" locations. Of course, if you're alone or with a blood relative, keep these notions to yourself.

- On the north side, cut through the passage in the 1919 Wrigley Building and follow the plaza to the enormous thing to the left of the Wrigley. Too big for its own good, you say? Too ostentatious, just too, too much? Well, you're fired. Mr. Donald Trump's self-named hotel and condo high-rise mushrooms up to nearly 1,200 feet, and that's before the spire. It replaces the unloved *Chicago Sun-Times* Building, which was meant to evoke a river barge and succeeded all too well. When complete, the Trump promises a multi-level plaza and walkway along the river. If you're there before the opening, you might have to detour via N. Wabash Ave.

- Cross N. Wabash Ave. and pause on the plaza in front of the once-landmark 1971 IBM Building, whose position has been, well, trumped. Directly across and below upper Wacker Dr., the Vietnam Veterans Memorial Plaza was completed in 2005. It lists names of those killed and has fountains and grassy areas. But one problem with the plaza is that it's not linked to the plazas on either side of the bridges. In fact, none of the plazas along the south bank—many with nice little summertime take-out cafes—are linked. For whatever reason, when the recent zillions were spent rehabbing Wacker Dr., no links were put in, meaning that trying to walk along the south bank is akin to surmounting a never-ending succession of dunes. Not fun, and anyway, the view's better from the north bank riverwalk.

- Cross N. State St. and you're in the midst of the landmark Marina City complex. Ignore the inappropriate Smith & Wollensky atrocity/steakhouse and focus on the timeless genius of architect Bertrand Goldberg. As fresh today as when they opened in the early 1960s, the towers are timeless. Always high-profile, they had a starring role in the 1980 Steve McQueen movie *The Hunter* when a speeding car shot out of the 15th floor of the parking garage and into the river.

- Once past N. Dearborn Ave., you can quickly pass the Westin Hotel and the former headquarters of Quaker Oats.

- Take the narrow walk in front of the 1914 building west of N. Clark St. that's now home to Encyclopedia Britannica and cross LaSalle St. The new 60-story building here at 300 N. LaSalle promises multiple layers of riverwalks when it opens in late 2008. But you still may have to dart around behind the gaudy little former headquarters of the company that made Suave, the cheap shampoo.

- Dart under the El tracks at N. Wells St. and leave the waters by entering the Merchandise Mart. Once the Marshall Fields warehouse and for many years the largest building in the world, it is home to showrooms of furniture and interior décor dealers and wholesalers. And you'll find water again at the Kohler showroom near the east entrance; the running waters may inspire a comfort stop. In fact, the Mart makes a good break with its bustling food court and fine, hotel-like lobby area. The almost-700-foot-long central corridor hums with activity weekdays but is dead weekends.

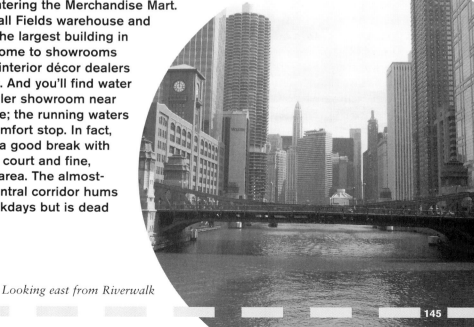

Looking east from Riverwalk

- Emerging at the west end, angle across N. Orleans St. toward the river and take the stairs down to the wondrous circular path that follows the curve of Wolf Point. Pause at one of the best-placed benches in the city and take in the split of the Chicago River. The South Branch heads off through a canyon of high-rises, while the North Branch meanders off with far less drama. Opposite, you can't help but be enthralled by the genius of the 333 W. Wacker Dr. Building, whose curving swath of green glass perfectly mirrors the river. Tour boats chug past and El trains rattle across the Lake St. Bridge. It's quite a scene.

- Follow the path along the North Branch. Try not to stare at the *Chicago Sun-Times* Building. When it was known as the Apparel Mart, it vied with the old *Sun-Times* building for the ugliest on the river. Maybe the paper should hire an architecture critic.

- Walk past the old railroad bridge that's now locked in the up position until somebody finds the wherewithal to tear it down. In the not-so-distant past, railroad tracks along the south bank served industrial sites all the way to the lake.

- Begin crossing the W. Kinzie St. Bridge, stopping after about 50 feet. Look down: this is the where one of the most tragi-comic episodes in Chicago's recent past occurred. Before dawn on April 13, 1992, the basements of buildings across the Loop began filling up with water. While officials suspected some sort of water main break, a reporter discovered what looked like a giant bathroom drain swirling down at the Kinzie Bridge. In the ensuing hours, the entire Loop was evacuated, scores of buildings were shut down, and $2 billion in damage was done to the underground guts of the Loop. Eventually the cause was sorted: crews installing new pilings for the bridge had caused a disruption in a tunnel under the river that was part of a little-known system of utility tunnels linking most of the buildings downtown. Privately built to carry coal and utilities, they had been abandoned decades before and mostly forgotten until water, complete with fish, filled up the basements of places like the Palmer House and the Board of Trade.

- During the peak of the flood, residents of the trapezoidal condos at the west end of the bridge sat drinking beer while city crews dumped huge boulders and mattresses into the swirling waters, where they vanished like so many stray hairs in a bathtub.

Back Story: Chicago's Bascule Trunnion

It sounds like the character in an Agatha Christie play, but bascule trunnion (or trunnion bascule) is the type of bridge most identified with Chicago. Basically a huge leaf (the bascule) sits on a giant axle (the trunnion) and simply rotates up and out of the way of river traffic. When sailboats and vessels in need of clearance navigate to or from the lake, the synchronized raising and lowering of the Chicago River bridges is almost operatic and one of the city's great—and free—spectacles.

- Walk south on N. Canal St. and angle over to the diminutive riverwalk in front of the rather pedestrian condo buildings at 333 N. Canal St. At the south end, curve around back to Canal St. and cross the tracks. With a constant cacophony of train bells and horns plus crossing gate bells, it's a train-spotter's opera down here.

- Walk up and east along W. Lake St. for about 200 feet and then take the utility access road behind the sturdy brick condo-conversion at 165 N. Canal St. Note the primo riverfront air rights available over the tracks between you and the river. But don't dwell on it and spoil the karma of those who currently have the views.

- At W. Randolph St. jog east again until you are on the riverwalk in front of the headquarters of the Boeing Co.

- Stop as you cross W. Washington St. (avoid becoming a hood ornament of a speeding cab, of course) and look east. On a clear day you can see the Frank Gehry-designed bandshell twinkling in the sun almost a mile distant—yet another reason to forgive the 558 percent it went over budget. Immediately south the old 1929 building of the long-gone and still-missed *Chicago Daily News* has easily the best plaza on the South Branch. Amidst its mannered charm are good views of its contemporary east across the river, the Civic Opera Building. Every tour guide that bobs past on a boat claims that the developer, Samuel Insull, wished the west face to resemble a throne, so I'll say it too.

- At Adams you can stop as the riverwalk continues past just a couple more cut-rate modern office buildings. Instead take a moment to appreciate the classic colonnaded lines of Union Station one block west. Wander inside the S. Canal St. entrance and go down the same stairs used for the landmark baby stroller scene in *The Untouchables*. The waiting area is airy and skylit, and also possibly doomed. An especially horrific proposal is floating around to crush Union Station under a huge tower. Given that the last time I was there, many benches had vanished and the train monitors were all broken, the cynic in me suspects the beginnings of a "see, no one uses it" argument.

- You can catch one of the many bus lines at Union Station or catch the El at stations beginning at Wells St.

CONNECTING THE WALKS

At the beginning of this walk, you can hook up with Walk 16 at either its start or its finish. At the end of this walk, cross over into the Loop and join Walk 17.

POINTS OF INTEREST

Bridgehouse and Chicago River Museum 376 N. Michigan Ave., 312-977-0227
Trump International Hotel and Tower www.trumpchicago.com

ROUTE SUMMARY

1. Begin at the mouth of the Chicago River, on the south bank just east of Lake Shore Dr.
2. Walk through the 170-foot-long tunnel under Lake Shore Dr.
3. On the west side, walk along the grass and tree-lined river bank.
4. At the Michigan Ave. Bridge, climb 20 steps and cross Lower Michigan Ave. to the base of the southwest tower of the bridge.
5. Climb to the upper level of the N. Michigan Ave. bridge and cross north.
6. On the north side, cut through the passage in the 1919 Wrigley Building and follow the plaza.

7. Cross N. Wabash Ave. and stay along the river.

8. Cross N. State St.

9. Once past N. Dearborn Ave. take the narrow walk in front of the building west of N. Clark St. and cross LaSalle St. Navigate around the new building to N. Wells St.

10. Dart under the El tracks at N. Wells St. and cut through the Merchandise Mart.

11. Emerging at the west end, angle across N. Orleans St. toward the river and take the stairs down to the circular path that follows the curve of Wolf Point.

12. Follow the path along the North Branch.

13. Cross the W. Kinzie St. Bridge.

14. Walk south on N. Canal St. and angle over to the diminutive riverwalk in front of the condo buildings at 333 N. Canal St. At the south end, curve around back to Canal St. and walk south.

15. Walk up and east along W. Lake St. for about 200 feet and then take the utility access road behind the brick condo-conversion at 165 N. Canal St.

16. At W. Randolph St. jog east again until you are on the riverwalk in front of the headquarters of the Boeing Co.

17. Walk along the river to W. Adams St.

18. At Adams, walk west one block and go in the S. Canal St. entrance of Union Station.

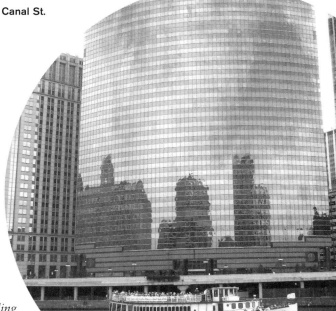

Tourist boat in front of the 333 Wacker Building

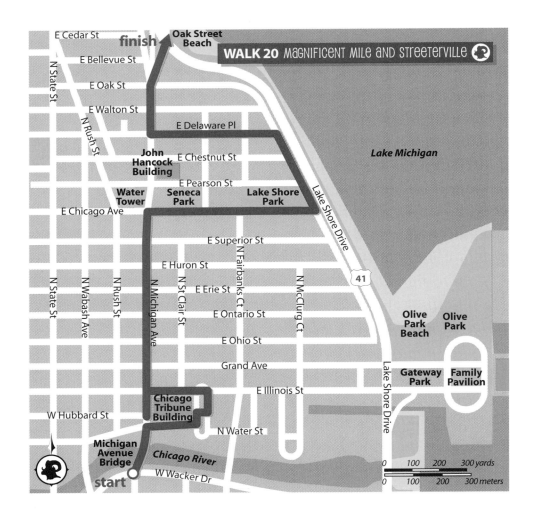

E Cedar St

finish

Oak Street
Beach

E Bellevue St

WALK 20 MagNiFiceNT Mile aNd Streeterville

E Oak St

N State St

E Walton St

N Rush St

E Delaware Pl

John
Hancock
Building

E Chestnut St

Lake Michigan

Water
Tower

Seneca
Park

E Pearson St

Lake Shore
Park

Lake Shore Drive

E Chicago Ave

E Superior St

E Huron St

N Fairbanks Ct

41

E Erie St

N McClurg Ct

N State St

N Wabash Ave

N Rush St

N Michigan Ave

N St Clair St

E Ontario St

E Ohio St

Olive
Park
Beach

Olive
Park

Grand Ave

E Illinois St

Lake Shore Drive

Gateway
Park

Family
Pavilion

Chicago
Tribune
Building

W Hubbard St

N Water St

Michigan
Avenue
Bridge

Chicago River

0   100   200   300 yards

start

W Wacker Dr

0   100   200   300 meters

20 MagnifiCent Mile and StreeterVille: rich rewards

BOUNDARIES: Oak St. Beach, N. Lake Shore Dr., Chicago River, N. Michigan Ave.
DISTANCE: 2 miles
PUBLIC TRANSIT: Numerous El and Bus lines stop near the beginning of the walk

For many it's their favorite urban walk in America, and with its flowers and architectural charms, the stretch of N. Michigan Ave. from the Chicago River north to Oak St. Beach is undeniably appealing. Known as the Magnificent Mile or Mag Mile or even Boul Mich, the street sucks in hordes of shoppers, for whom it may be the ultimate fantasy strip mall. But look past the commercialism and you'll find many slices of Chicago's past and discover the fabric that makes the city so interesting. And as a reward, you get to squish sand between your toes.

- Start your walk at the south end of the N. Michigan Ave. Bridge. The four 1928 bridge towers (which many think would make great *pied-á-terres*) each sport a panel depicting a key moment in Chicago's early history. On the southwest *The Defense* shows the 1812 Fort Dearborn massacre replete with tomahawk-wielding braves (and note the confusing profusion of brass plates in the sidewalk that show the supposed outline(s) of the original fort, which would have been over 50 feet below). On the southeast, *Regeneration* shows a graft-free version of reconstruction after the fire. Cross the bridge. On the northwest tower, *The Pioneers* shows John Kinzie, for once not selling booze to the natives, and on the northeast, *The Discoverers* shows landmark names Louis Joliet and Jacques Marquette busy discovering.

- Walk over to the plaza in front of the 401 N. Michigan Building, where there is much to see. First, gaze west at the Wrigley Building. With its two parts, you could say the building is the place to "double your pleasure, double your fun." The primary part with the clock tower dates from 1919, and given its presence, few realize that the 1924 addition to the north is actually 50 percent larger. Now spin around and confront the moose. Sculpted from old chrome auto bumpers by John Kearney in 2002, it has a commanding presence and is one of dozens of chrome critters that Kearney has placed on Chicago streets through the years.

- Walk east across the plaza, passing "Studio 5," the now *de rigueur* streetside studio of NBC5 (a.k.a. WMAQ-TV). It's actually a bit of a kludge, as the station has its newsroom in the NBC Tower 500 feet east, but needed a location closer to butt-cheek-mooning pedestrians. If the anchors look rather, well, frigid in winter, it's because they must scoot across the plaza to appear on camera. Note that WGN Radio has its own streetside studio in the southwest corner of the Tribune Tower on the north side of the plaza. And if you moon daytime hosts Kathy O'Malley and Judy Markey, they'll probably like it.

- Continue on the plaza east until you get to the richly landscaped N. Cityfront Plaza Dr. There's some nice public spaces here, and as you walk north, you're in the heart of one of the last major commercial areas to be developed near N. Michigan Ave. Were you to continue east, the Riverwalk on the north bank of the Chicago River plunges deep into condo land, but because of the Chicago Spire construction doesn't smoothly meet up with the lakefront.

- Turn west on E. Illinois St. On the right, you'll see the new Avenue East high-rise, which has been grafted onto the back of the landmark Intercontinental Hotel. You might notice a painted scrawl reading "Wyland" on the bit of the hotel's east wall that still shows. That's all that's left of the huge and beloved mural painted by the noted whale-artist. No doubt if Avenue East gets the wrecking ball before the Intercontinental (likely given today's "efficient" construction techniques), the Wyland mural will be rediscovered to much acclaim.

- On your left is the Tribune Tower. This 1934 addition defers to the Gothic 1923 original, but shares the same collection of rocks from famous places embedded in the walls. When you reach N. Michigan Ave., follow the Tribune building around to the entrance of the McCormick Tribune Freedom Museum. This recent and rather curious institution is meant to celebrate the First Amendment, although it really reinforces the bland Republican values the *Chicago Tribune* usually espouses (just wait for the gauzy shot of a kid with a gun in the intro film). However, the whitewash is saved for the display on Col. Robert McCormick, the crackpot owner and publisher of the *Tribune* from 1910 to 1955. Although a strict isolationist (he thought Hitler should have his way with England in 1940), he also pioneered foreign coverage in American newspapers, sending reporters hither and yon (and badgering them to bring home rocks for his walls).

Back Story: Streeterville

The neighborhood east of the Mag Mile is named Streeterville in memory of Capt. George Wellington Streeter, a skipper whose skills as a seaman were so limited that he needed a first mate named Gilligan. While sailing from Milwaukee to the Caribbean in 1886, he came up a bit short when he ran aground in the mud off what is today's E. Chicago Ave. However, once on damp land, Streeter proved far more wily as a developer. For the next 30 years he invited builders to dump debris around his boat, helping to form much of what is today's Streeterville. Although the city and established developers tried to drive him off, he successfully sold deeds to others who shared his pioneering spirit.

- Back out on Michigan Ave., look for the stairs leading down to the gothic horrors of Lower Michigan Ave. Descend, and cut over to the northwest corner with W. Hubbard St. Avoid the pigeon poop and plunge into the Billy Goat Tavern. "Legendary" is too simplistic for this decades-old haven for beer-swilling media types. By day, there's often a few too many tourists, but you can enjoy the charms of bartender Jeff Magill. By night, journalists who've staved off liver failure can still be found. Take time to read the walls—including in the bathroom—and pick up a copy of Rick Kogan's touching reminiscence *A Chicago Tavern*.

- Return to daylight on Michigan Ave. and walk north. With its lavish plantings and many attractive storefronts, N. Michigan Ave. lives up to its Magnificent Mile billing (a moniker which dates to the 1940s when one of Chicago's great real estate hustlers, Arthur Rubloff, was looking for a way to peddle this then-developing part of town). The half-mile from the Tribune Tower to E. Chicago Ave. has some of the most expensive retail rents in the country. Pick your own highlights on the stretch, but one worth honoring is the Crate & Barrel store at 646. Its bright exterior—like a box for its clean-lined goods—is perfectly symmetrical and white. But what makes it worth acclaim is that instead of building a Brobdingnagian terror that the zoning would have allowed, the owners stuck to four stories in honor of the Mag Mile's traditional and now vanishing scale. Side note: no cynic can resist the charm of the millions of tiny white lights lining the avenue during the holidays.

- At E. Chicago Ave., stop. Try not to become roadkill for the hordes of young girls learning the proper way to drink tea while maxing out their parents' credit cards at American Girl Place. On the northwest corner is the genuine Water Tower, the 1869 castellated Gothic survivor of the fire. Although iconic, it's ironic that it was just a big pipe to relieve water pressure on the 1866 pumping station east across Michigan. Inside there are often short-term exhibits by local artists and photographers. The surrounding landscape has been substantially upscaled, although the new "chairs" seem mostly designed to keep anyone—especially non-shoppers—from getting too comfy. Inside the boxy and long decommissioned pumping station, the city has an excellent tourist office.

- Walk east on Chicago Ave. The 1902 firehouse at 202 picks up design cues from the Water Tower and really just needs a Dalmatian to complete the cliché. (And note the heroic posie-growing efforts of the firefighters.) At N. Mies van der Rohe Way (more on him in a bit), the Museum of Contemporary Art (MCA) initially looked like something that crawled out from under Albert Speer's bed, but in the more than 10 years it's been here, the harsh metal panels have taken on a sort of warm sheen, and the seemingly Everest-like front steps have become a popular meeting point, with loungers arrayed like hams in a deli.

- Continue east to Lake Shore Park while enjoying the tweets and whistles of the songbirds chirping it up in the gardens behind the MCA. A rare bit of open space in this high-rent district, the tennis courts are packed with residents and med students from Northwestern Memorial Hospital, which is located in the blocks south of E. Chicago Ave. Having honed their skills at the best prep schools, the competition is as fierce as that for a patient with full insurance coverage.

- Angle across the park northeast to inner N. Lake Shore Dr. and walk one block north to E. Chestnut St. Ahead of you the condo buildings at 860 and 880 look like hundreds of others you've seen, right? Well, these were the first buildings built (1949–1951) by Mies van der Rohe in his International style, and they've spawned thousands of often ham-fisted copies since. Mies continued to hone his stark steel and glass visual language in the years that followed from his studio at the Illinois Institute of Technology on the South Side (see Walk 10).

- Walk west on E. Delaware Pl., noting the additional apartments (1953–1956) by Mies at 900 and 910, until you reach N. Michigan Ave. To your southeast—in case you didn't notice—is the John Hancock Center, the sloping slab in Miesian style that combines retail, commercial and residential space in one 1969-vintage municipal icon. Pass down through the sunken plaza (ignoring the tourists over-eating chain-fare at the Cheesecake Factory) and take the 40-second ride to the 94th-floor Observatory. This one beats its more popular rival in the Sears Tower because the lines are shorter, it's cheaper, from here you can take in the entire Loop skyline with the Sears Tower in it and there's a nifty open-air area where you can enjoy the roar of the city.

- Back on terra firma, walk north on N. Michigan Ave. The building on the southeast corner with E. Walton Pl. has regained the name it was christened with in 1929: the Palmolive Building. However, it's still known to many as the Playboy Building, the name Hugh Hefner had erected in huge letters across the apex during the years (1965–1989) when the magazine was based here. Today this Art Deco charmer has been converted to condos (and there's no truth to the rumors that the units in the old photo studio spaces still reek of silicon).

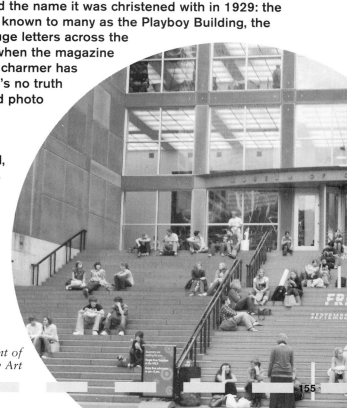

- Directly across Walton from the Palmolive Building is the Drake Hotel, which continues its role as Chicago's most traditional hostelry (it opened in 1920). If there's a big blow off the lake and your cockles need warming, settle in for a bowl of signature Bookbinder soup at the Coq d'Or restaurant.

- The Mag Mile ends at E. Oak St.; celebrate with a beach frolic. Cross Oak and take the walk that runs under

Crowds waiting in front of the Museum of Contemporary Art

Lake Shore Dr. You emerge onto the perfect crescent of sand that is Oak St. Beach. Chicago is one of very few cities where you can dart away from your desk at lunch, scamper to the shore and be back at your desk in time for another Powerpoint presentation. In summer, Oak St. Beach has a nice little ephemeral cafe, plenty of competitive volleyball matches and lots of beautiful people.

- From Oak St. Beach you can walk north three-quarters of a mile to North Ave. Beach with its fantasy steamship bathhouse and quieter expanses of sand. The hook-shaped breakwater there has fabulous views back to the Mag Mile.

- Numerous bus lines pass the intersection of E. Oak St. and N. Michigan Ave.

CONNECTING THE WALKS

From North Ave. Beach you can continue one mile north to where Fullerton Dr. meets the lake and hook up with Walk 23. Or from Oak St. Beach, walk south almost a mile on the concrete walk along noisy Lake Shore Dr. and link up with Walk 16 at Navy Pier. One final option: join Walk 21, which starts at N. Michigan Ave. and E. Oak St.

POINTS OF INTEREST

Billy Goat Tavern 430 N. Michigan Ave. (lower level), 312-222-1525

McCormick Tribune Freedom Museum 445 N. Michigan Ave., 312-222-4860

American Girl Place 111 E. Chicago Ave., 312-943-9400

City of Chicago Tourism Office Water Tower Pumping Station 163 E. Pearson Ave., 877-244-2246

Museum of Contemporary Art 220 E. Chicago Ave., 312-280-2660

John Hancock Center Observatory 875 N. Michigan Ave., 312-751-3681

Coq d'Or Drake Hotel, 140 E. Walton Pl., 312-787-1431

route summary

1. Start at the south end of the N. Michigan Ave. Bridge.
2. Walk over to the plaza in front of the 401 N. Michigan Building.
3. Walk east across the plaza.
4. Turn left on N. Cityfront Plaza Dr.
5. Turn left on E. Illinois St.
6. Take Michigan Ave., and go down the stairs leading down to Lower Michigan Ave.
7. Go to the northwest corner with W. Hubbard St.
8. Return up to N. Michigan Ave. and walk north.
9. Turn right on Chicago Ave.
10. Cut across Lake Shore Park northeast to inner N. Lake Shore Dr.
11. Walk north on Lake Shore Dr.
12. Turn left on E. Delaware Pl.
13. Turn right on N. Michigan Ave. and walk north to Oak St. Beach.

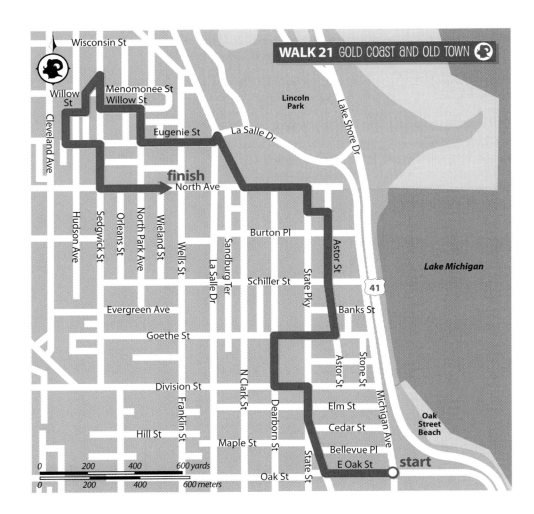

Wisconsin St

Willow St

Menomonee St
Willow St

Cleveland Ave

Eugenie St

La Salle Dr

Lincoln Park

Lake Shore Dr

finish
North Ave

Hudson Ave

Sedgwick St

Orleans St

North Park Ave

Wieland St

Wells St

Sandburg Ter

La Salle Dr

Burton Pl

Astor St

Lake Michigan

Schiller St

State Pky

Evergreen Ave

Goethe St

Banks St

41

Division St

N Clark St

Dearborn St

Astor St

Stone St

Elm St

Michigan Ave

Oak Street Beach

Franklin St

Cedar St

Hill St

Maple St

State St

Bellevue Pl

E Oak St

start

Oak St

0   200   400   600 yards

0   200   400   600 meters

21 GOLD COAST AND OLD TOWN: THE COLOR OF MONEY

BOUNDARIES: **W. Wisconsin St., N. Astor St., E. Oak St., N. Cleveland Ave.**
DISTANCE: **2½ miles**
PUBLIC TRANSIT: **151 Sheridan Bus. Numerous other lines stop close by.**

The Gold Coast has always been just that: the place where the folks with the gold live near the coast. Since the 1880s it has been home to some of Chicago's wealthiest families, and much of the neighborhood feels timeless. The nightlife on nearby Rush St. also seems timeless, but maybe that's just plastic surgery. Just north, Old Town was once a modest worker's enclave, but time and gentrification have turned it into a lovely yet exclusive place where finding something to buy for under seven figures means sharing a floor. Walks here are rich in history, beauty and charm—but not necessarily all three at once.

● **Start your walk at the intersection of N. Michigan Ave. and E. Oak St. This walk takes you through Chicago's ritziest areas, so you may want to look the part. Oak St. is the exclusive enclave for those who find the Mag Mile just so common. It's lined with boutiques, and you'll actually see plenty of Lexus's—or better—double-parked, engines running and drivers waiting stoically. You can smell the exfoliate in the air as you pass by the Marilyn Miglin Institute, the ultra-high-end cosmetic boutique. This is pure Oak St. (and this block is named in the proprietor's honor).**

● **Turn north on N. Rush St. At 1028 you won't miss Gibson's, the reigning steakhouse of the Gold Coast and singles playground for the moneyed class of a certain age. The steaks are thick and juicy, and that might describe some of the people at the bar. If you're male and a millionaire, you may be lucky to escape with your hairplugs.**

● **Gibson's fittingly overlooks a little patch of land where Rush St. meets N. State St. known as the "Viagra Triangle." The name is an apt tribute to the generations of lounge lizards who have prowled these blocks looking for hoots. There have been nightclubs here since the 1940s, and Rush St. was the place for slightly more mature** singles to frolic since the days when "playboy" meant a man in a smoking jacket with a pipe. Disco had its day here, and generations have caroused in its nightclubs. Yet this isn't where you'll find hipsters and scenesters; the nightclubs of the moment are far to the west. Instead, the area generically known as Rush Street serves those who want conversation with their foreplay as opposed to an exchange of cold hard cash.

- For a classic pop or a toot, stop into Jilly's at 1007 N. Rush. The whole Sinatra vibe is in over-drive here, right down to the rows of celeb pix on the wall. It's a fine place for a martini while you groove to the piano bar; just don't reflect on the fact that Frank was already dead when it opened.

- Turn west on W. Division St. The next block is a somewhat more desperate version of Rush St., with hawkers outside of old standards like Butch McGuire's and Mother's. Cries of "Try sex on the beach!" greet you after dark.

- Escape the squalor by turning north on N. Dearborn St. Typical of the Gold Coast, it is lined with a mix of vintage charmers and all-together nastier modern concrete high-rises. The unassuming four-flat at 1239 was the home of Ernest Hemingway and his first wife Hadley Richardson in 1921. Married that year, the couple set up house in an apartment they found "dark and depressing" in what was then a dodgy part of town. Earning money through newspaper writing, Hemingway and Hadley left for Paris at the end of the year—pulled abroad by hopes of new writing opportunities and the promise of no Prohibition.

- At W. Goethe St., turn east. Note that in Chicago it's not *Ger-ta* as the German philosopher would have pronounced it but—we're not making this up—*Go-thee*. Sometimes it's hard to wash the prairie out of the city. On the northeast corner with N. State St., the Ambassador East Hotel has been a gracious retreat since 1927. It's home to the Pump Room, a classic lounge and restaurant that has maintained its appeal for decades. For once, the rows of celebrity photos in the foyer are authentic. Hitchcock fans will know that this is the hotel where Cary Grant made nice with Eva Marie Saint before he went off to his date with the cropduster in *North by Northwest*.

- Continuing east you'll feel the air become more rarified as you near N. Astor St. When Chicago's elite were chased out of their Prairie Ave. mansions by encroaching industry and vice, many settled on this half-mile-long street in what was then countrified seashore. Through the 1940s they built a huge variety of mansions and exclusive homes, most of which survive today and make an Astor St. stroll endlessly rewarding. A few highlights south to north follow: 1308-1312, the surviving troika of what had been four 1887 rowhouses show a cohesive sculptural quality. Architect John Wellborn Root was so pleased with the results that he moved into 1310. At 1345, the current owners maintain the street's high standards with luxuriant plantings; at 1355, animals of all kinds can be found in the stone details on this uncommon-for-Chicago 1914 Georgian. A tantalizing glimpse of the courtyard reveals a seahorse cavorting in a fountain. The Charnley House, 1365, was an early work of Frank Lloyd Wright, who cheerfully bragged that it was the "first modern house." At times it's open for tours.

- Cross E. Schiller St. and continue north. The highlights continue: 1406 is an imposing mansion that was built for Joseph T. Ryerson, Jr., son of the man who started the Chicago firm that pioneered the use of stainless steel. With kitchen trends going in for the industrial look, were the house built today it would be a lot grander. 1425 is a huge gray Georgian that was built for the industrious William Kerfoot, who the day after the Chicago fire reopened his store in a shack with a sign that read EVERYTHING GONE BUT WIFE, CHILDREN AND ENERGY. 1500, a massive 1893 mansion, was doubled in size in 1927.

- Just past 1524, look for the alley and take a left. Note how many of the exposed pavers are still blocks of oak. To the north is the 1880 Queen Anne mansion for the archbishop of the Chicago Roman Catholic Diocese. Ignoring the whole

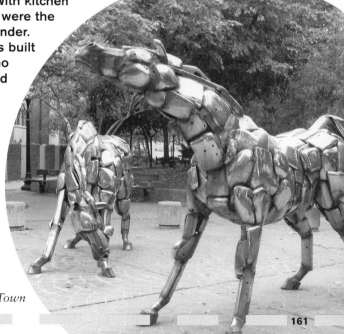

Horse sculpture by John Kearney, Old Town

"vow of poverty" debate for moment, you'll note that the current resident likes fresh-off-the-vine tomatoes.

- Jog up N. State Pkwy. to North Ave. and turn west. The 1555 N. State Pkwy. building on the southwest corner was the premier apartment building on the Gold Coast when new in 1912. Each floor had but one or two residences.

- At the corner with N. Clark St. cross north and stop by the Chicago History Museum, the new name for a generation that finds the old name, Chicago Historical Society, off-putting. It's a fascinating look into the city's attic, and traces the vast and endlessly entertaining threads of the city's past (think *The Sopranos* multiplied by 1,000).

- Where the six lanes of N. La Salle St. cross Clark, find your way west across the asphalt desert into the heart of Old Town. There's an immediate calm as you hit W. Eugenie St. that only intensifies as you cross N. Wells St.

- Old Town only came by its name after World War II, when the residents of the somewhat Bohemian community of old worker's cottages and rehabbed houses formed a strong neighborhood organization to promote and protect what until then had been cleverly called North Town. Having helped the area navigate through decline in the 1950s and 1960s followed by rapid improvement in the 1970s, the organization continues today and sponsors a wildly popular art fair in June. For a good intro to the neighborhood, stop and ponder the four houses at 215-225 W. Eugenie St. Built in 1874, they slipped under the wire before post-fire reforms banned wooden houses like this. Each has taken a different course in the decades since. Nos. 215 and 217 have elaborate carvings and their original form; 219 has suffered from some bad DIY stairs; 221 was replaced by a typical brick three-flat; and 225 gives the neighborhood an upscale finger with a fortress-like wall in front.

- Turn around and face north. You're looking at Crilly Court, a private development built over a 10-year period from 1885. Note the proud stone columns marking the north and south entrances to the street. Details here abound, but take special note of the four houses on the east side named after the developer's children. On the west side, the pleasing harmony of the stone Queen Anne façades is counteracted if you step west to the alley and see the riot of backside variations that have occurred over the years.

- Walk north on N. North Park Ave. two blocks and turn west on W. Menomonee St. About 150 feet after you pass N. Orleans St. there's an alley on the north side. The otherwise non-descript, tiny house on the northwest corner is a rare surviving example of the one-room houses that were constructed for fire survivors in 1871. They were designed to be carried by wagon and might be considered the FEMA trailers of the day—only built significantly better. The south side of the street has a mixed bag of wooden row-houses that give a good idea of what the city looked like in the 1870s—if you can look past the over-restoration on some and under-restoration on others.

- Turn north on N. Sedgwick St. On the east side there's a long row of modern houses that were built at the time Ogden Ave. was removed in the early 1970s. Ridding the area of this major thoroughfare accelerated the renovation and, yes, gentrification of Old Town. Note how owners of these "modern" homes are applying classical details to them with abandon.

- After about 250 feet, look for a pedestrian area running sharply southwest along the alignment of the old Ogden Blvd. Try to resist the urge to mount the chrome-bumper horse sculptures by John Kearney (although we must admit we rode one until we were saddlesore at a boozy party here a few years back). The sidewalk empties into a cute little plaza with tables designed for chess. Just west at the corner of N. Hudson Ave. and W. Menomonee St., the building, still bearing the sign of the long-closed Schmidt Metzgerai, recalls the era when North Town was the province of German laborers.

- Do a little jig first east onto N. Fern Ct. and then west onto W. Willow St. and south onto pint-sized N. St. Michael's Ct. You've skirted the 1971 Midwest Buddhist Temple, which has a lot of parking for the devout. Where St. Michael's meets W. Eugenie St. you can see the reason for its name: St. Michael's Church, which has an interior rich with ornamentation provided by its Bavarian flock in the 1800s.

- One block east at the corner with N. Sedgwick St. is Twin Anchors, a timeless rib joint and bar with leather booths and but one glowing newspaper clip in the window— from 1982.

- After dark and as close to midnight as you can make it, venture south to W. North Ave. and east to N. Wieland St. There on the corner is a shrine to authentic Chicago taverns, the Old Town Ale House. Catering to an eclectic and idiosyncratic crowd, it has been reinvigorated just enough recently to spare it from death. Once inside, before you know it, it'll be 4 AM outside (5 AM Sunday mornings).

- Numerous busses on N. Clark St. will take you north or south. Or ride the 72 North bus west to the Red Line El stop at North/Clybourn. If you've been to the Ale House, just take a cab.

POINTS OF INTEREST

Marilyn Miglin Institute 112 E. Oak St., 800-662-1120

Gibson's 1028 N. Rush St., 312-266-8999

Jilly's 1007 N. Rush St., 312-664-1001

The Pump Room 1301 N. State Pkwy., 312-266-0360

Charnley House 1365 N. Astor St., 312-915-0105

Chicago History Museum 1601 N. Clark St., 312-642-4600

Twin Anchors 1655 N. Sedgwick St., 312-266-1616

Old Town Ale House 219 W. North Ave., 312-944-7020

ROUTE SUMMARY

1. Start at the intersection of N. Michigan Ave. and E. Oak St.
2. Walk west on Oak St.
3. Turn right on N. Rush St.
4. Turn left on W. Division St.
5. Turn right on N. Dearborn St.
6. At W. Goethe St., turn right.
7. Turn left on N. Astor St.

8.   Just past 1524 N. Astor St., look for the alley and take a left.

9.   Turn right up N. State Pkwy. to North Ave. and turn left.

10. At the corner with N. Clark St. turn right and walk north.

11. Cross Clark and N. La Salle St. to W. Eugenie St. and walk west.

12. Turn right on N. North Park Ave.

13. Turn left on W. Menomonee St.

14. Turn left on N. Sedgwick St.

15. After about 250 feet, look for a pedestrian area running sharply southwest along the alignment of the old Ogden Blvd. The sidewalk empties into a little plaza.

16. Do a little jig first right onto N. Fern Ct. and then left onto W. Willow St.

17. Turn left on N. St. Michael's Ct. and walk south.

18. Turn left on W. Eugenie St. and walk east.

19. Turn right on N. Sedgewick and walk south to W. North Ave.

20. Turn left and walk east to N. Wieland St.

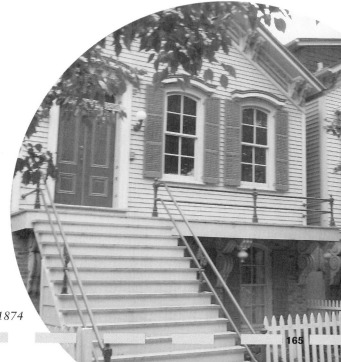

W. Eugenie St. cottages dating from 1874

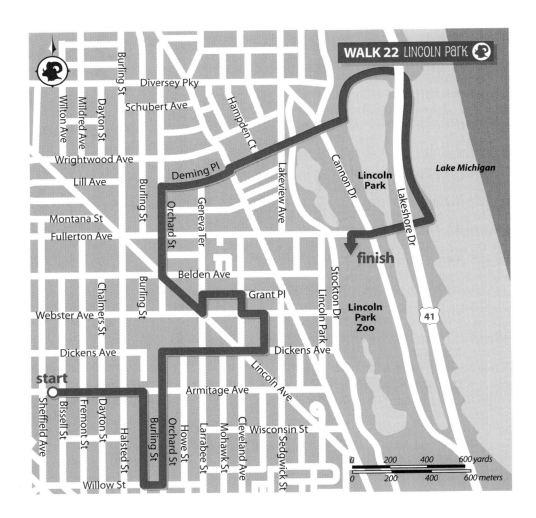

Burling St
Diversey Pky
Schubert Ave
Hampden Ct
Wilton Ave
Mildred Ave
Dayton St
Wrightwood Ave
Deming Pl
Lill Ave
Lakeview Ave
Cannon Dr

Lincoln Park

Lake Michigan

Burling St
Orchard St
Geneva Ter
Montana St
Fullerton Ave
Lakeshore Dr

Belden Ave
Chalmers St
Burling St
Grant Pl
Stockton Dr
Lincoln Dr
Lincoln Park

finish

Webster Ave

Lincoln Park Zoo

Dickens Ave
Dickens Ave

Lincoln Ave

Armitage Ave

start

Sheffield Ave
Bissell St
Fremont St
Dayton St
Halsted St
Burling St
Orchard St
Howe St
Larrabee St
Mohawk St
Cleveland Ave
Wisconsin St
Sedgwick St

Willow St

41

| 0 | 200 | 400 | 600 yards |
| 0 | 200 | 400 | 600 meters |

22 LINCOLN Park: NOTHING exceeds LIKe excess

BOUNDARIES: W. Diversey Pkwy., Lake Michigan, W. Willow St., Oz Park
DISTANCE: 4¼ miles
PUBLIC TRANSIT: Brown Line El to Armitage stop

Lincoln Park is sort of like the old Certs ad or the Saturday Night Live fake ad for Shimmer: It's a park! It's a neighborhood! It's a park! It's a neighborhood! No, you're both right! For the record, the neighborhood does take its name from the park, which covers 1,200 acres and stretches from North Ave. in the south 6 miles north to the end of Lake Shore Dr.; most people, though, think it only covers the widest area, which stretches north to Diversey. It's packed with attractions, including miles of walking paths, beaches, a great zoo and much more. In fact, it's packed with things many people don't know about, like hundreds of bodies at the south end where there was a cemetery before the park was started in 1864 (many remains were moved, but the efforts were lackadaisical, as is clear every time a hole gets dug for a project). The neighborhood, Chicago's most popular, runs west of the main patch, although its borders tend to expand exponentially when the definition is left to Realtors ("Lincoln Park West" seems to mean anything east of Iowa). It's filled with beautifully restored vintage housing and includes a huge range of shops, cafes, restaurants, and bars. You can spend days walking here; the tour below covers some classic sights and includes a few surprises.

- Start your walk on W. Armitage Ave. under the El tracks. If it's a hot day, why wait for relief? Start off fresh at Annette's Homemade Italian Ice on the corner with N. Bissell St. The ice cream and other frozen treats are fresh with flavors that pop. And just in case you didn't know you weren't, say, in Berwyn, there are soy-based doggie treats for the upscale vegan pooch.

- Armitage from N. Halsted St. to N. Racine Ave. is one of Chicago's most upscale streets; the strip mall as it were for one of the most expensive neighborhoods in the city. As such there's plenty of services. Need a bit of handmade writing paper? All She Wrote has sheets of paper costing dollars each (and they're beautifully worth every penny). Need a cowl neck sweater? (Is it the 1970s again?) Intermix has 'em for $268. Need your 400th pair of shoes? Try Lori's. Need a snack? Charlie Trotter has one. . . . Okay, we got carried away. But for a mere $125 the legendary Trotter will make you dinner at his famed restaurant, set in twin brick two-flats as carefully land-scaped outside as the food is arranged on the plate inside. If you linger out front, the valet will give you a menu to take away—no reheating needed.

- As you're strolling or sauntering—nobody does anything as mundane as walk here—look up and down streets such as N. Dayton St. The canopy of trees over the street and timeless brick homes go a long way to explaining the inherent appeal of this and other parts of Lincoln Park (and for that matter the North Side).

- Cross N. Halsted Ave. and turn south on N. Burling St. Prepare yourself for a shock: you've found ground zero for Chicago's nouveau riche (and that includes some old riche who are acting pretty darn nouveau). About 100 yards along and on the west side you'll encounter something that could have been dropped in from France—or Mars. It's the $40-million, 20,000-square-foot mansion of Richard Parrillo, a very rich insurance agent. It sits on the site of the former Infant Welfare Society of Chicago (now ensconced a few miles west where infant needs are somewhat greater). And though it's the biggest, it's by no means the only Leviathan on the block, because a size war has broken out on N. Burling and neighboring N. Orchard and N. Howe sts.

- Going south, house after new house has been built right up to its property lines. And because this part of town has no alleys, one after another of these new beasts has a cut-out drive that slopes steeply down into a Land Rover-sized garage. Any sense of street life is lost in this Verdun-in-the-city, or as Blair Kamin, the *Chicago Tribune* architecture critic wrote: "The doors to these sunken garages look like the gates of hell."

- Try to keep your lunch down and turn east one block on W. Willow St. and then north again on N. Orchard St. The same juxtaposition of grand old and gross new is at work here. Celebrate the vintage homes that enjoy their place in the city, right down to the basketball hoops over the street. But as you think about the unfortunate consequences of cutting taxes for the rich, keep your spirits up by counting how many times you spot a comical miscue like a supposed architectural pillar mounted above a garage door. These folks may have money, but they don't have taste.

- Cross W. Armitage Ave. and follow the pedestrian extension of Orchard along the front of Lincoln Park High School. On Saturdays the farmers market here is one of the best in the city. Turn east on the pedestrian portion of W. Dickens Ave. (there was a lot of urban renewal here in the 1970s) and after you pass N. Howe St., walk on for another four blocks.

- Turn north on N. Hudson Ave. Walk slowly, as you're looking for 2121, one of the very oldest homes in the city. The 1871 fire reached its limits near here, and the owner of the house at the time, a cop named Richard Bellinger, saved his home by throwing water on the roof (although some more flavorful versions of the story cite cider as the flame retardant). Today the house has a new foundation, but otherwise is close to its 1860s appearance.

- Walk the rest of the block north on Hudson and turn west on W. Webster Ave., then north one block on N. Cleveland Ave. Turn west on diminutive W. Grant Pl. The Contemporary Art Workshop is the studio of John Kearney, the artist responsible for the delightful animal sculptures made from chrome bumpers that are found all over town (see Walks 20 and 21). Fancy a beaver or maybe a giraffe? You can get one here.

  From the west end of Grant Pl., head south one block on N. Geneva Terrace. This is the heart of Chicago Landmark-designated Mid-North District, with its profusion of late 19th-century Italianate and Queen Anne styles. As you walk you might realize that you aren't in Kansas anymore, because after two blocks you'll hit the northeast corner of Oz Park. It's named in honor of Lyman

N. Orchard St. McMansions, Lincoln Park

Frank Baum, who wrote all 14 of his Wizard of Oz books while living in Chicago (see Walk 29 for details).

Few realize that the movie is based on *The Wonderful Wizard of Oz*, the first of many books. Fewer know that the ninth book in the series, *Tik-Tok of Oz*, centers on a shipwrecked girl from Oklahoma and her mule. Obviously Hollywood made the right choice for adaptation. Imagine your own Yellow Brick Road as you wander the east end of the park. Look for the large statues of the Tin Man, Scarecrow, Cowardly Lion and Dorothy and Toto. You can even cavort in the Emerald Garden.

● Okay, if it's a hot day you're entitled to one screech of "I'm melting!" Otherwise exit the park the way you entered, and walk northwest on N. Lincoln Ave. This stretch has something for everybody. Sterch's is a classic old-time saloon that's been there forever, as have many of the genial regulars. Look for the carrot over the door. On the east side of the street, the fabled Victory Gardens Theater has their Greenhouse, which is literally the place where new talent and plays are nurtured. It's just one small cog in Chicago's muscular theater scene.

● After one block turn north on N. Orchard St. North of you is the vast complex of Children's Memorial Hospital, which is moving to join the even vaster complex of Northwestern Memorial Hospital in Streeterville. What's left here is as sure to fall prey to jackals (a.k.a. developers) as a hapless wildebeest in a National Geographic special. After you cross W. Fullerton Ave., look for the Chateauesque trio of homes starting at 2424. Built in 1895, they were especially grand for this middle-class area.

● Turn east on W. Deming Pl. The north side of this gently curving street has a medley of fine 1890s homes broken just occasionally by the 1960s version of the contemporary Orchard St. horror: the evil 4+1. Built by the hundreds across the north side, they crammed dozens of apartments into spaces that once held a single-family home or maybe a two-flat (see 546 on this block as an example). Happily, construction was so shoddy that they should start collapsing any day now. Otherwise, enjoy the gracious elegance at 632, 612 and 526, among others.

● Cross N. Clark St. and as you walk east on Deming, you'll notice a lot of construction. That's because Columbus Hospital, which once occupied a major chunk of the south side of the street, has already fallen prey to the jackals, and in its place is "2520 Lincoln Park," the largest and tallest (39 stories) condo development locally in some time.

- Cross N. Lakeview Ave. and go under the N. Stockton Dr. pedestrian bridge (where Jake and Elwood hid near the end of *The Blues Brothers*) and walk straight east to North Pond, the much-acclaimed restaurant overlooking—you guessed it—the North Pond in Lincoln Park. Chef Bruce Sherman does wonders with classic Midwestern ingredients in this Arts and Crafts gem. Sunday brunch and lunch are big in warm months.

- Follow the curving path north and east, crossing N. Cannon Dr. Amble over to Diversey Harbor and follow the waterside path north and east yet again. That whack you hear in the distance is the Diversey Driving Range, north of the parking area. If hitting the long ball is not your forte, there's also a sweet little miniature course, although it sadly lacks a little windmill.

- Cross under Lake Shore Dr. When you reach the main lake path, look for *A Signal of Peace Monument*. There's a real dignity to the expressions of both the rider and the horse, and unlike the Grant Park stallions (see Walk 6), this is not an ad for Cialis.

- Walk south along the lake for about a half mile. This area has received the controversial new shoreline treatment, as well as dozens of new trees. Many decry the new walls as dull and lacking the features of the old ones, although the main feature of the replaced walls was broken concrete.

- When the Theater on the Lake comes into view, head inland on Fullerton Dr. (The theater has evolved into a legitimate venue; in summer, some of the leading theaters in town stage performances there.) Watch out for careening SUVs as you navigate the LSD off-ramps; at rush hour cars get backed up and soon Lincoln Parkers pretty much drive like maniacs, with phone clamped to an ear with one hand while the other simultaneously blows the horn and flips the bird in all directions.

- Cross the bridge over the rowing lagoon. There's usually lots of people fishing here, especially in fall when they're hoping to nab salmon, trout and perch. To the north you'll get a glimpse of the beige Notebaert Nature Museum, which is exactly what the name implies (you can find out what lives in the ponds, if you must) and which struck visitor gold after it installed a walk-with-the-butterflies exhibit.

● Dodge past the people waiting to park in the southern extension of N. Cannon Dr. and look for the gated entrance to the Alfred Caldwell Lily Pool on the south side of Fullerton. Something of an overlooked gem, the pond here is the namesake of landscape architect Alfred Caldwell, who was a contemporary of Frank Lloyd Wright. Prairie style is used throughout to create an idealized version of a Midwestern stream, replete with waterfall, pavilion and artfully arranged rocky outcrops. Like so much of the Park District, the area suffered greatly from neglect beginning in the 1950s. It was even renamed the Rookery and made an adjunct to the zoo, where people could see whatever birds happened to fly by. In 2000 a massive renovation began that restored the brilliance of Caldwell's design, and it has now been designated a National Historic Landmark. Circling the meandering paths around the ponds—which do indeed have lilies—is a fine way to end this walk.

● From the lily pond, it is easy to catch one of the many bus lines that pass the park. Or you can visit the Lincoln Park Zoo, which is immediately south and is rightfully one of the most popular attractions in the city. You can even make faces at a gorilla.

CONNECTING THE WALKS

You can link the lakefront portion of this walk with Belmont Harbor and Walk 26 in the north by walking three-quarters of a mile north from Diversey Harbor. Or head back out to the lake and walk 1 mile south to link up with Walk 20 and the lakefront to the south.

POINTS OF INTEREST

Annette's Homemade Italian Ice 2009 N. Bissell St., 773-868-9000

Intermix 841 W. Armitage Ave., 773-404-8766

All She Wrote 825 W. Armitage Ave., 773-529-0100

Lori's Shoes 824 W. Armitage Ave., 773-281-5655

Charlie Trotter's 816 W. Armitage Ave., 773-248-6228

Sterch's 2238 N. Lincoln Ave., 281-2653

Victory Gardens Theater Greenhouse 2257 N. Lincoln Ave., 773-871-3000

North Pond 2610 N. Cannon Dr., 773-477-5845

Notebaert Nature Museum www.chias.org, 2430 N. Cannon Dr., 773-755-5100

Lincoln Park Zoo www.lpzoo.com, 2001 N. Clark St., 312-742-2000

route summary

1. Start on W. Armitage Ave. under the El tracks.

2. Walk east and turn right on N. Burling St.

3. Turn left and walk east one block on W. Willow St. Turn left again on N. Orchard St.

4. Cross W. Armitage Ave. and follow the pedestrian extension of Orchard along the front of Lincoln Park High School. Turn right on the pedestrian portion of W. Dickens Ave. and after you pass N. Howe St., walk on for another four blocks.

5. Turn left on N. Hudson Ave.

6. Turn left on W. Webster Ave., then right one block on N. Cleveland Ave. Turn left on W. Grant Pl.

7. From the west end of Grant Pl., turn left and head south one block on N. Geneva Terrace to Oz Park.

8. Exit the park the way you entered and walk northwest on N. Lincoln Ave.

9. After one block turn right on N. Orchard St.

10. Turn right on W. Deming Pl.

11. Cross N. Lakeview Ave., go under the N. Stockton Dr. pedestrian bridge and walk straight east to North Pond.

12. Follow the curving path north and east, crossing N. Cannon Dr. Walk to Diversey Harbor and follow the waterside path north and east yet again.

13. Cross under Lake Shore Dr. and walk south along the lake for about a half mile.

14. Head inland on Fullerton Ave.

15. Enter the Alfred Caldwell Lily Pool on the south side of Fullerton.

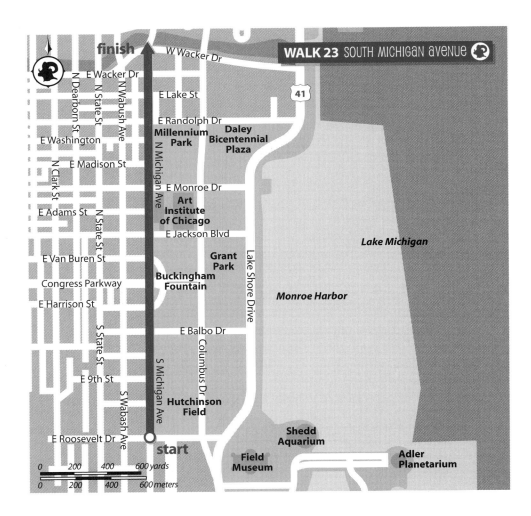

finish

W Wacker Dr

E Wacker Dr

N Dearborn St

N State St

N Wabush Ave

N Michigan Ave

E Lake St

E Randolph Dr

E Washington

E Madison St

N Clark St

E Monroe Dr

E Adams St

N State St

E Jackson Blvd

E Van Buren St

Congress Parkway

E Harrison St

Millennium Park

Daley Bicentennial Plaza

Art Institute of Chicago

Grant Park

Buckingham Fountain

Lake Shore Drive

Lake Michigan

Monroe Harbor

41

E Balbo Dr

Columbus Dr

S State St

S Michigan Ave

E 9th St

S Wabash Ave

Hutchinson Field

E Roosevelt Dr

start

Field Museum

Shedd Aquarium

Adler Planetarium

| 0 | 200 | 400 | 600 yards |
| 0 | 200 | 400 | 600 meters |

23 SOUTH MICHIGAN AVENUE: THE SOUL OF CHICAGO

BOUNDARIES: **Chicago River, Grant Park, E. Roosevelt Rd., Michigan Ave.**
DISTANCE: **1½ miles**
PUBLIC TRANSIT: **Green, Orange and Red Line El to the Roosevelt stop**

Though relatively short, this walk takes in the soul of the city, the stretch of Michigan Ave. between Roosevelt Rd. and the river. This has always been the city's front porch. It's where Montgomery Ward showed he had a soul by vowing to save the lakefront from development. It's where the city found its cultural soul in great music and art. And it's where the city questioned its soul during days of protest and violence. As you make your way north, don't be surprised if some parts of this walk touch *your* soul.

● Begin your walk surrounded by what seem to be many souls, 106 to be exact. Near the southwest corner of Grant Park at S. Michigan Ave. and E. Roosevelt Rd. is *Agora*, one of the edgiest works of art to grace public land in Chicago since the Picasso came to the Loop. The headless, roughly cast torsos on legs represent the crowds who worship or hate leaders in time of war, said the artist, Polish-born Magdalena Abakanowicz in 2006, when she was 76. The torsos shuffle about in a crowd, their rust staining the concrete blood-red.

● Beginning at E. 11th St. and Michigan Ave., you'll pass several buildings that are part of Columbia College, a fast-growing arts institution that emerged from humble origins and began hitting its stride in the 1980s. Its departments are scattered in buildings across the South Loop. On the northwest corner with 11th, the Music Center is home to a highly regarded graduate program in music composition for the screen. Among the famous grads of Columbia is Janusz Kaminsky, a cinematographer who works with Steven Spielberg, and who won Oscars for *Schindler's List* and *Saving Private Ryan*.

● At E. 8th St., the Chicago Hilton and Towers literally looms large. For many years after it opened as the Stevens Hotel in 1927, it was the world's largest hotel, with over 3,000 rooms. (Sending out all those room-service breakfasts in the morning was a feat that would stymie NASA today.) Conrad Hilton bought it in 1945 and slapped his

BACK STORY: DAYS OF RAGE

On August 26, 1968, at the peak of the Democratic National Convention, several thousand hippies, yippies and people just sick of the Vietnam War gathered in front of the Chicago Hilton, where most of the presidential candidates were staying. Despite their numbers, the protestors were outnumbered by the Chicago Police, who had already shown a propensity to beat anyone in sight during the previous nights in Lincoln Park. No one is exactly sure what sparked what was later termed by investigators as a "police riot," but soon blue-helmeted cops were bludgeoning protestors, journalists, conventioneers, and even each other. In one bit of low comedy, several injured people were taken to the suite of presidential candidate Eugene McCarthy, only to have the door suddenly burst open and Chicago cops run in and beat up everyone in sight. The chaos in Chicago meant the Democrats didn't come back for a convention until 1996, and it ensured the election of Richard Nixon.

name on the place; in the 1980s it received a lavish remodeling that cut the number of rooms down to a mere 1,600. Much has happened here through the years, but the most infamous moment happened right in the lobby on August 26, 1968, when the Chicago police chased protestors inside and beat the crap out of them. (See sidebar.)

● The Blackstone, another grand hotel, is just across E. Balbo Ave. from the Hilton. It opened in 1910 and represents a truly extravagant version of the French Beaux-Arts style, from the soaring Mansard roof to the wedding cake of a base. And like its neighbor, the Blackstone also played a role in presidential politics: in 1920 the Republicans had their convention in Chicago, and in an era when presidential candidates were actually selected at the convention, found themselves hopelessly deadlocked. Finally the weary bosses, exhausted from booze and cigars, decided on Warren Harding, whose sole credential for the job was that he looked presidential. A reporter said he'd been chosen in a "smoke-filled room," and a political cliché entered the lexicon. (Harding turned out to be a disaster as president, with an administration caught up in scandals that wouldn't be equaled for over 80 years. He was also known for his philandering ways, a rep he shared with another president 40 years later who also often stayed at the Blackstone: John F. Kennedy.) The Blackstone today has been lavishly rehabbed, and is now part of the Marriott empire.

- Mid-block, the Spertus Institute of Jewish Studies documents 5,000 years of Jewish faith and culture, and gives it a distinctly Chicago spin. In 2007 it moved from rather drab quarters to a stunning new building right next door. The 10-story glass façade is composed of 726 pieces in 556 shapes. It has an evocative texture that from some angles suggests flames.

- At the corner of E. Harrison St., the Museum of Contemporary Photography is run by Columbia College and features changing shows of some of the best work being done today. East across Michigan Ave. are some of the most colorful details of Grant Park (see Walk 6).

- On the north side of Congress Pkwy. is another masterpiece of Chicago architecture, the Auditorium Building. The combined talents of Louis Sullivan and Dankmar Adler created this 1889 masterpiece, with its trendsetting mix of a rusticated stone base and polished limestone above. The 4,200-seat Auditorium Theater is dramatic even when dark, and has perfect acoustics. Even Frank Lloyd Wright, who treated praise as if it was water and he was in a lifeboat adrift at sea, said it was "The greatest room for music and opera in the world—bar none." Owned by Roosevelt University for many decades, there are grand spaces throughout the building. It's worth stopping in to see what's open for view.

  Note the arcade on the Congress Pkwy. side. It was created out of retail space after the road was widened as part of the 1950s and 1960s orgy of expressway construction.

- The very next building north is another cultural treasure. The Fine Arts building houses over 150 artists, performance groups, and support businesses like violin repairers and sheet-music dealers. The ground-floor Artists Cafe doesn't quite live up to the promise of its iconic marquee, but much of the rest of the building is a delightful surprise.

- North of E. Van Buren St., you are in the very heart of the city-designated Michigan Boulevard Landmark District, which runs from E. 11th St. to E. Randolph St. The official designation says it is "as if some of the best of Chicago architecture gathered along the lakefront and posed for a group photo." You can get a full perspective of this clan at several points on Walk 6 in Grant Park.

- The block north of E. Jackson Blvd. has another worthy cultural attraction. The 1904 Santa Fe Center was home to its architect Daniel Burnham. Within the sparkling white terra-cotta exterior is a sun-drenched interior light well. The Chicago Architecture Foundation is based here, and their tours by land and water are highly recommended. Next door is the Symphony Center, which includes the Burnham-designed Orchestra Hall. It's hailed both for its flawless acoustics and its house band, the Chicago Symphony Orchestra.

- Finally something on the east side of the street other than manicured gardens and statues: the Art Institute of Chicago. Amidst the thousands of works and miles of corridors is one work that relates perfectly to your walk: *Nighthawks*, Edward Hopper's 1942 study of urban ennui. A huge new Modern Wing built on the Columbus Dr. side of the Art Institute will increase gallery space by a third and include a soaring pedestrian bridge to Millennium Park.

- For details on the bright lights of Millennium Park on the east side north of E. Monroe St., see Walk 16. On the west side of N. Michigan Ave., plan a pause at the Chicago Cultural Center in the block north of E. Washington St. Built as the city's library in 1897, today the imposing walls shelter a range of galleries with ever-changing exhibitions (this is always a good refuge when the weather takes a wrong turn), a decent cafe, and a city tourist information office. Revel in the rich detailing, including luminescent mosaics and the Tiffany-domed grand staircase.

- On the southwest corner of N. Michigan Ave. and E. Randolph St., trade the Cultural Center's high art for low life. Descend the steps to what is today called Millennium Station and you find the last stop of Jake Lingle, who was gunned down here in 1930. The *Chicago Tribune*'s ace crime reporter, Lingle probably got a little too close to his sources (who included Al Capone), as he was rubbed out right here by a gunman who vanished into the crowd. After his death it was discovered that Lingle's bank account exceeded his $65 weekly salary by a factor of 1,000. A lot of money, but is that fair value for a soul?

- North of Randolph, the east side of Michigan is mostly lined with the bland 1970s development known as Illinois Center, whose overall esthetic puts the last four letters in "banal." Wander in and you may find it hard to escape from the low-ceilinged passageways lined with fast-food joints and chains.

- On the west side, the major buildings of note before you reach the river are the Hard Rock Hotel, a striking ebony, green and gold shaft that was built in 1929 as the Carbon and Carbide Building, and the 1923 360 N. Michigan Ave. building, which mirrors the bend in the river and has a beautifully restored lobby.

CONNECTING THE WALKS

This walk links up with several others. At the north end you can continue right up Michigan Ave. on Walk 20, or join Walk 19 along the Chicago River. Not far away, Walk 17 covers the Loop. At E. Randolph St., Walk 16 starts in Millennium Park and ends at Navy Pier. The oft-mentioned Walk 6 covers parts of Grant Park along S. Michigan Ave. before heading south to the Museum Campus and beyond. Finally, Walk 13, covering the South Loop and Near South Side, begins at E. Roosevelt Rd.

POINTS OF INTEREST

Columbia College www.colum.edu, 600 S. Michigan Ave., 312-663-1600

Spertus Institute of Jewish Studies 610 S. Michigan Ave., 312-322-1700

Museum of Contemporary Photography www.mocp.org, 600 S. Michigan Ave., 312-663-5554

Roosevelt University www.roosevelt.edu, 430 S. Michigan Ave., 312-341-3500

Auditorium Theater www.auditoriumtheater.org, 50 E. Congress Pkwy., 312-922-2110

Chicago Architecture Foundation www.architecture.org, 224 S. Michigan Ave., 312-922-3432

Chicago Symphony Orchestra www.cso.org, 220 S. Michigan Ave., 312-294-3000

Art Institute of Chicago www.artic.edu, 111 S. Michigan Ave., 312-443-3600

Chicago Cultural Center 78 E. Washington St., 312-744-6630

route summary

1. Start at E. Roosevelt Rd. and walk north on S. Michigan Ave. to the Chicago River.

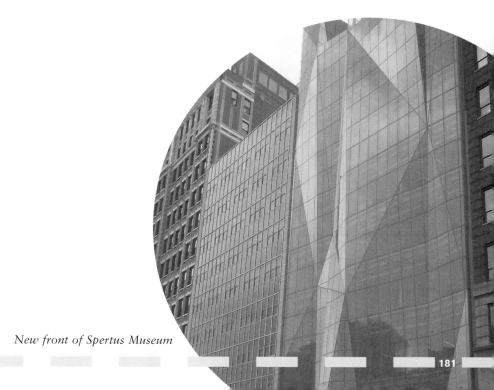

New front of Spertus Museum

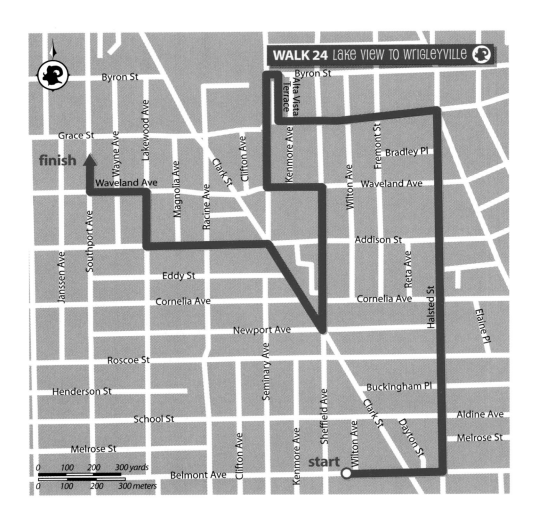

Byron St

Byron St

Alta Vista Terrace

Grace St

finish

Wayne Ave

Lakewood Ave

Magnolia Ave

Clark St

Clifton Ave

Kenmore Ave

Fremont St

Bradley Pl

Waveland Ave

Wilton Ave

Waveland Ave

Southport Ave

Racine Ave

Addison St

Janssen Ave

Eddy St

Cornelia Ave

Reta Ave

Cornelia Ave

Halsted St

Elaine Pl

Newport Ave

Roscoe St

Seminary Ave

Henderson St

Buckingham Pl

School St

Sheffield Ave

Clark St

Aldine Ave

Melrose St

Dayton St

Melrose St

Clifton Ave

Kenmore Ave

Wilton Ave

start

Belmont Ave

0   100   200   300 yards
0   100   200   300 meters

BOUNDARIES: **W. Grace St., N. Halsted St., W. Belmont St., N. Southport St.**
DISTANCE: **3 miles**
PUBLIC TRANSIT: **Brown and Red Lines El to Belmont stop**

A roughly 1-square-mile chunk of the North Side, with Clark St. as its diagonal spine and running north from Belmont Ave., may hold more fun for more people than any other part of the city. The stretch along Halsted carries the cheerful badge "Boystown," while up by Addison, Wrigley Field anchors the most concentrated nightlife strip in Chicago. Of course like anywhere, there's good, there's bad and yes, there's ugly (especially when talking about the Cubs), but on a walk through here you can't help but see numerous joints that will lure you back after dark.

- Start your walk at the newly rebuilt Belmont El stop. Almost under the tracks, Berlin has been a dance club since long before some of the patrons were born. Refreshingly unadorned, it caters to a mixed crowd of people whose persuasion ends in sexual (homo, hetero, trans, etc.). Madonna night here is like all-you-can-eat pasta night at the Olive Garden: perfectly targeted at the clientele.

- Walk east on W. Belmont St.—where the crowd is like that in Berlin, only with better skin-tone—and you'll see the bright new home of ComedySportz, where teams of comedians compete for laughs. This especially muscular form of improv comedy is only the latest iteration of the wide-ranging, free-associating hunt for hilarity practiced at Second City.

- Passing the intersection with N. Clark St., there's often unintentional street theater at the Dunkin' Donuts, where a hardcore crowd makes good the epithet "Punkin' Donuts."

- Turn north on N. Halsted St. If you were wondering what neighborhood you were in, the upthrust, phallic and rainbow-rimmed street standards waste no subtlety in proclaiming "Boystown!" For decades, Halsted St. north of Belmont has been Chicago's gay neighborhood, and it's not slowing down. Day and night it's a genial carnival where camp is the new conservative.

- The eponymous Roscoe's (note the cross street) is the mainstream gay bar of the street, the kind of place you'd take your mother after coming out of the closet. Nearly opposite, Sidetrack has a glitzy new vibe that belies its old sobriquet: Sidetrash. The rooftop deck seats 350. And right nearby are two places where you can snatch a snack: Pie Hole Pizza if you want to eat out (most people prefer the 18-inch large), and Nookies Tree, which has classic coffee-shop fare, including hot lunch specials.

- One block north at the intersection with W. Newport Ave., the Chicago Diner celebrates what in Chicago is the ultimate alternative lifestyle: vegetarianism. Look for dishes like Polenta Fiesta and the enticingly named Scrambled Tofu Delight.

- Relatively discreet by Halsted St. standards, Batteries Not Included caters to the kind of crowd who giggle so hard at the thought of a vibrator that it becomes moot. For a much harder sell, cross the street and go up a block to Cupid's Treasures, which has four rooms of any device, potion or accessory you can think of—and that's just in the Nun Fantasy Department.

- Cross W. Addison St. (the street of tears, more in a bit), and stop at—we are not making this up—the old Sexauer Garage at 3640. Say what you want about Whole Foods (Whole Paycheck anyone?), but the company did a bang-up job restoring the Sexauer-family-run grease-monkey joint for a new century. Just look at that winged wheel on the façade. The complex includes the glam new Center on Halsted, a vibrant community center for lesbian, gay, bisexual and transgender (LGBT) people of all ages. There are programs on constantly, so stop in and see what's up.

- Across the street, you can buy a vintage frock and support a good cause at the Brown Elephant Resale Shop. Thousands of items from trash to treasure are on sale here; proceeds go to the nearby Howard Brown Health Center, which treats the ever-growing numbers of uninsured and under-insured.

- If the Kit Kat Lounge had a subway grate out front, Madame X in her Marilyn persona could repeat the iconic *Seven Year Itch* scene ad nauseam. But such regular blows aren't missed inside at this transgender female-celebrity impersonator club, which appeals to an audience ranging from middle-aged suburbanites to the campiest denizens of Boystown.

- At W. Grace St. it's time to bid the pleasures of Halsted St. adieu for the mainstream delights of Wrigleyville. Walk five blocks west to a truly unique Chicago street. Turn north on N. Alta Vista Terrace, a one-block wonder that recreates London rowhouses. Twenty units on each side of the street use a variety of materials and details to obscure the fact that they're really just one building. The two sides diagonally mirror each other. The units were meant for workers when built in 1904, but today are quite fashionable, if rather tiny. This was the city's first Historic District.

- At the north end of Alta Vista, swing around to the west and return south on the paved alley with the broad adjoining grassy strip. Up until the 1970s, there were train tracks on the strip that connected up with the El North near Wilson Ave., as the El actually used to carry freight at night. The tracks here served the heavy industries once found across Lakeview during a time when the phrase "heavy industry" meant more than "moving the plasma TV to dust around it."

- Continue to W. Waveland Ave. and Wrigley Field. Say what you want about the Chicago Cubs, but they have the best stadium in baseball. There are stories aplenty about the place—most involving the phrase "lovable losers"—so we'll just say

Boystown street sign

this: on a sunny afternoon, hanging out with friends, watching a game here is one of Chicago's great experiences.

- Go east on Waveland. Where N. Kenmore Ave. butts in is where people hang out waiting for homers—the more astute doing so during actual games. At N. Sheffield Ave. turn south. The bar on the corner, Murphy's Bleachers, is something of a legend, but for us it's legendary for jacking up prices on game days and employing bartenders who constantly demand tips. Actually, that's typical of most of the bars around here on game days.

- Sheffield used to be lined with humble three-flats, where on game days a few friends might get together on the rooftops and enjoy some bad but cheap domestic beer while watching the game. Today almost every building here is topped by a private club where members get together and enjoy some bad but expensive domestic beer while they yak into their cell phones. Given the unquenchable thirst for tickets (they are lovable losers, after all), the Cubs' management and the private clubs have reached a sort of détente.

- Cross W. Addison St. (the trail of tears story is coming . . .) and spare a thought for the Chicago White Sox. Their owners are the ones who decreed that the few bars and whatever street life there was around the old Comisky Park be replaced by parking lots when the former new Comisky Park (presently branded for U.S. Cellular, but next week?) was built in 1991. Boneheads.

- Where Sheffield meets N. Clark St., make the 270-degree turn and confront your fate: ahead lies one of the greatest concentrations of bars in Chicago, and a no-brainer of a case study for any MBA student who wants to combine education with drinking (hmmm . . . where do we apply?). Over the three long blocks from here to W. Grace St., there are dozens of bars—mostly on the west side of street—supporting the supposition that to make a killing running a bar in Chicago, all you need do is a) locate near Wrigley Field, b) buy a lot of TVs and c) give your place a vaguely Irish name. In fact, of the following names, guess which ones aren't actually bars here: Blarney Stone, Irish Oak, Mullen's, Houndstooth, Full Shilling, Casey Moran's, Dark Horse and Buggered Leprechaun. Okay, only the last one is fake.

Mostly undistinguished—and less than 10 years old—these bars pack 'em in game or no game. And the success has lured other bars in Chicago, such as Lincoln Park's charming John Barleycorn, to open mob-sized versions here lacking any of the charms that made the originals so delightful. Fortunately, amidst the mediocrity there are a few places of true character: If you can overlook the post-game posers, the Wild Hare has been a reggae hangout since 1986. The I.O., which is the hip name for the ImprovOlympic, is a legendary improvisational comedy bar. And up by Grace St., the Gingerman has a fine beer selection and avoids drinking the Cubs Kool-Aid.

● Rather than walk the entire Clark St. strip, turn west at Addison St. and escape to one of Chicago's finest neighborhood bars. But first we owe you a story: in 2007, when the Cubs by some twist of fate—or goat—got into the post-season, we were walking by Wrigley on one of the nights they were playing Arizona out of town. Wrigleyville was swarming with cops in case Cubs fans became so over-stimulated by victory that they would run out and burn down a fake Irish bar. A pair of policemen were nearby, and this is what we overheard. Cop One: "Pretty dead here, huh?" Cop Two: "Nothing's gonna happen, Addison's just a trail of tears for Cubs fans." Actually we have one more Cubs note: Addison St. is named for a British physician, Dr. Thomas Addison, who discovered a form of anemia. Hmmm . . .

● Three blocks west of Clark at N. Lakewood Ave., Guthrie's Tavern has been a welcoming hangout since 1986 (it's named for one of the owner's dogs back then). It has real character, board games by the dozen, and lots of cute little tables where you can enjoy the long list of good beers. There's not a poser or posturer in sight, but there is an always genial batch of locals. If you need a fourth for Monopoly, you'll likely be in luck.

● You may want to end at Guthrie's, but it's worth pushing on just a tad more. Walk north on Lakewood and then two blocks west on W. Waveland Ave. to N. Southport Ave. Although the name was hyped by Realtors in the 1980s in an effort to take then-mutton (Lake View) and dress it up like lamb (Wrigleyville), the efforts weren't really necessary, as this part of Chicago has an inherent and unassuming charm that has universal appeal (ignoring the recent tumorous growths of fill-in McMansions).

- Walk north on Southport, letting yourself be drawn like a mayfly to the marquee of the Music Box Theater. Inside this 1929 classic, there's a Moorish fantasy of a movie palace. The films range from classic to off-beat to foreign, and are hand-picked. Enjoying one here is a treat, and after all you've seen on your walk, you can use the time at rest to decide where you're going back to after the lights come up. (If it's a revival of *The Quiet Man*, you get no credit unless you go back to the Kit Kat Lounge and demand one of the ladies do a full Maureen O'Hara.)

- To leave the neighborhood, the Red Line El stop for Addison is about three-quarters of a mile east, the Brown Line El stop for Southport under half a mile south. The 22 Clark bus runs around the clock.

POINTS OF INTEREST

Berlin 954 W. Belmont Ave., 773-348-4975

ComedySportz 929 W. Belmont Ave., 312-733-6000

Dunkin' Donuts 3200 N. Clark St., 773-477-3636

Roscoe's 3356 N. Halsted St., 773-281-3355

Pie Hole Pizza 739 N. Halsted St., 773-525-8888

Nookies Tree 3344 N. Halsted St., 773-248-9888

Chicago Diner 3411 N. Halsted St., 773-935-6696

Batteries Not Included 3420 N. Halsted St., 773-935-9900

Center on Halsted 3656 N. Halsted St., 773-472-6469

Brown Elephant 3651 N. Halsted St., 773-549-5943

Kit Kat Lounge 3700 N. Halsted St., 773-525-1111

Murphy's Bleachers 3655 N. Sheffield Ave., 773-281-5356

Wild Hare 3530 N. Clark St., 773-327-4273

ImprovOlympic 3541 N. Clark St., 773-880-0199

Gingerman 3740 N. Clark St., 773-549-2050

Guthrie's 1300 W. Addison Ave., 773-477-2900

Music Box 3733 N. Southport Ave., 773-871-6604

route summary

1. Start your walk at the Belmont El stop.
2. Walk east on W. Belmont St.
3. Turn left on N. Halsted St.
4. Turn left at W. Grace St., walk five blocks west to N. Alta Vista Terrace and turn right.
5. At the north end of Alta Vista, swing around to the west and return south on the paved alley and continue to W. Waveland Ave.
6. Turn left on W. Waveland Ave.
7. At N. Sheffield Ave. turn right.
8. Where Sheffield meets N. Clark St., make a 270-degree turn and go north on Clark.
9. Turn left at Addison St. and go three blocks.
10. Turn right and walk north on N. Lakewood Ave.
11. Turn left on W. Waveland Ave. and go two blocks west to N. Southport Ave.

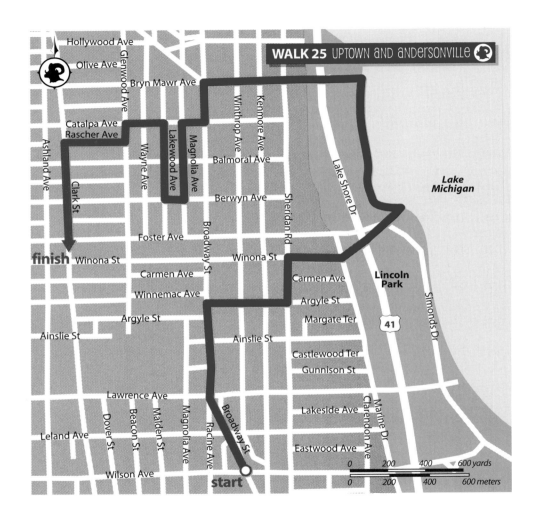

Hollywood Ave

Olive Ave

Glenwood Ave

Bryn Mawr Ave

Catalpa Ave

Rascher Ave

Ashland Ave

Clark St

Wayne Ave

Lakewood Ave

Magnolia Ave

Winthrop Ave

Kenmore Ave

Balmoral Ave

Berwyn Ave

Sheridan Rd

Lake Shore Dr

Lake Michigan

Foster Ave

Broadway St

finish Winona St

Winona St

Carmen Ave

Carmen Ave

Lincoln Park

Winnemac Ave

Argyle St

Margate Ter

Argyle St

Ainslie St

Ainslie St

41

Simonds Dr

Castlewood Ter

Gunnison St

Lawrence Ave

Dover St

Beacon St

Malden St

Magnolia Ave

Racine Ave

Broadway St

Lakeside Ave

Marine Dr

Clarendon Ave

Leland Ave

Eastwood Ave

Wilson Ave

start

0   200   400   600 yards

0   200   400   600 meters

25 UPTOWN AND ANDERSONVILLE: A TALE OF TWO CITIES

BOUNDARIES: **W. Bryn Mawr Ave., Lake Michigan, Wilson Ave., N. Clark St.**
DISTANCE: **3¾ miles**
PUBLIC TRANSIT: **Red Line El to Wilson stop**

In the 1920s, Uptown was a thriving entertainment district on the North Side. It was often compared to New York City, and just so that nobody missed the connection, it named its main artery Broadway. Meanwhile Andersonville, the neighborhood north of Foster Ave. and west of the El, upheld the values of its large Scandinavian population by staying tidy and not venturing far from the trim shops of Clark St. Today things have changed. Uptown fell on hard times, its bright lights extinguished by urban decay and an influx of poor people after the war, while Andersonville was discovered by new generations of discerning Chicagoans. Although gentrification may be finally bringing stability to Uptown—and lighting some of those lights—Clark St. thrives in Andersonville, which with its array of shops and lovely homes may be the most livable of the city's neighborhoods.

- Start your walk at W. Wilson Ave. and N. Broadway. You're in the heart of Uptown, the gritty North Side neighborhood that—like Brazil and Heather Graham—always seems on the verge of something great. Walk north on Broadway and you'll see the reality: improvements in fits and starts and a diverse street population of people at every stage—and station—in life. If you arrived by El, you'll note that the station is rather larger and more complex than most; when Uptown was at its peak in the 1930s, the El here was part of a rail system that had frequent trains going as far as Milwaukee. Today Skokie is your last stop.

- Head north on N. Broadway. At 4707 there are signs of upswing: the terra-cotta façade is a carnival of characters, all restored to their cartoonish best. Just north, Borders Bookstore is a bright light on the street, valiantly peddling books while it waits for long-rumored retail company in the long-discussed Wilson Yards complex set for south of W. Wilson Ave. One complication is that Uptown is covered by two aldermen: Helen Shiller, an old "progressive" whose 46th Ward—gerrymandering aside—generally covers the area south of Wilson, and the developer-friendly Mary Ann Smith, whose 48th Ward goes north from Wilson. Note which ward in Uptown looks better.

- At the intersection of Broadway and W. Lawrence Ave., stop and take in three enormous theaters still standing from a time when Uptown was the entertainment center for the North Side. Just south at 4746 N. Broadway, the 1918 Riviera Theater is fairly restrained compared to its later neighbors. It's now used for concerts. Over at 1106 W. Lawrence Ave., the 1926 Aragon Ballroom has more Moorish fantasy than you'll find in Spain. It too is now a concert venue. Finally, occupying a good chunk of the northwest block, the Uptown Theater is the grandest of them all. Its interior is another Spanish fantasy, this time Baroque. The Uptown has had a troubled life in recent years; it's so huge (almost 4,400 seats, second-largest in the United States) that plans for modern use have been elusive, but so grand inside that no one can bear to see it go. Blue tarps, á la post-Katrina New Orleans, are part of an effort to prevent further deterioration.

- Just south of the Uptown Theater, the Green Mill lives up to the promise of its iconic signage. It truly was a haunt of Capone and company during prohibition (ask to see the scrapbook behind the bar), and there are secret passages in the basement. Today it stays vibrant with some of the city's best live jazz and the fabled poetry slams on Sundays. There once was a bar named Green Mill, that never got around to going downhill . . . Boo! Get off the stage, loser!

- On the northeast corner, Demera Ethiopian opened to great acclaim in 2007, and brings African cuisine, art and music to Uptown.

- A tad north of the Uptown Theater, the Annoyance Theater presents entertainment that would have been unthinkable back when thousands were packing the Uptown to see family-friendly fare like 1927's *King of Kings*. The raucous shows, which include *Co-ed Prison Sluts* and *President Bush is a Great Man*, have launched the careers of actors like Beth Cahill and Amy Sedaris.

- As you near W. Argyle St., you'll leave Chicago for Southeast Asia. At the head of W. Argyle St., the Thai Grocery is not much to look at, but the sacks of rice and elaborate silver servers in the windows hint at what's inside.

- Turn east on Argyle. The jungle of signs reveals that you've reached the heart of the North Side's Asian community. Vietnamese, Cambodians, Laotians, Thais, and Chinese crowd the streets speaking a gaggle of languages as they transform themselves into new Americans. Storefronts hold simple cafes selling Pho noodles, groceries with exotic herbs found nowhere else in town, pharmacies with traditional remedies and stores with mundane but meaningful goods from home. Vietnamese are in the majority, as this was an official settlement area for refugees who found their way to America after the war.

- After three blocks, turn north on N. Sheridan Rd. Many of the once-grand apartment buildings are faded here, and the streets definitely have resisted the gentrification of neighboring areas. This is partly a legacy of the state's decades-old policy of dumping mental health patients in homes here, with little oversight.

- If Uptown is a melting pot, then the melting pot's melting pot is Big Chicks. Named by the owner Michelle Fire for the nickname she acquired backpacking in India, the crowd here includes lesbians, gays, straights and those unwilling to be classified at all. It gives new meaning to laid-back, and on Sundays its wonderful vibe is fully on display when a vast free buffet draws regulars as well as neighborhood old-timers who relish the free weenies.

- At W. Winona St., turn east to the lake and cross into Lincoln Park at N. Marine Dr., noting the welcoming little plots of posies tended by neighbors. Follow park paths north and east, crossing under Lake Shore Dr. on W. Foster Ave. Ahead and to the north lies Foster Ave. Beach, a real find that's spoken of in whispers by regulars lest the mobs farther south

The Green Mill, Uptown

hear the word. Much more mellow than Montrose or North Ave. beaches, the deep swath of sand here is often uncrowded. Refresh yourself at the beach house, which features some rather lush native gardens as well as deli food a few cuts above average.

● Walk north along the fairly unadorned lakefront for about half a mile to the W. Bryn Mawr Ave. underpass and head west into one of the North Side's quaintest little neighborhoods. You'll immediately see the vast quadruple-Y-shaped bulk of the Edgewater Beach Apartments. This 19-story pink fantasy was once part of the much larger Edgewater Beach Hotel complex to the south. Built in an era when people couldn't travel far for their beach vacations, the Edgewater was a luxury resort whose era faded when Lake Shore Drive was extended through its front yard in the 1950s and you could get a cheap flight to Florida.

● The three blocks of W. Bryn Mawr Ave. between N. Sheridan Rd. and Broadway comprise a delightful commercial strip with some interesting architecture and shops. At 1021, the Manor House is an unusual example of baronial luxury in Chicago. Originally there were only six apartments in the 1908 building, and they came with amenities like billiard rooms. The rents in the 1920s were about $250 per month, a huge amount when the average wage was less than half that. On the north side of the street across N. Kenmore Ave., the Belle Shore Apartment Hotel shines under a sheath of restored green terra-cotta that's alive with Egyptian figures.

● Pass under the El and you may get a whiff of something not normally sniffed near the El. Flourish Bakery Cafe is living up to its name, with a panoply of treats that are just like mom used to make, with one critical difference: you don't need a nostalgic filter to think they taste good. Pecan sticky bun, anyone?

● Cross the five-way circus that's the intersection of Bryn Mawr, N. Broadway and N. Ridge Ave., and stop into two stores that reward browsers: Kate the Greats is a tidy little bookstore with new, used and rare titles; around the corner, Alchemy Arts is lined with hundreds of potions, lotions and other aromatic substances used for occult and metaphysical practices. Here's your chance to load up on saltpeter.

● For spirits who have gone mainstream, walk south on Broadway until the Gothic mass of St. Ida's Church looms into view. St. Ida's opened in 1927 when the Chicago

Roman Catholic Archdiocese was at the peak of its powers and the legendary Cardinal Mundelein was literally building what he thought would be an empire for the ages. When plans for the church were presented, the cardinal "suggested" that French Gothic, the style of Notre Dame and Chartres, would be nice. The architect, Henry Schlacks, complied and did him one better by working the letter "M" into the ornamentation. Inside, richly carved wood continues the Gothic detailing.

- Stroll west on W. Catalpa Ave. for one block; the church and associated buildings line the entire south side of the street. At N. Magnolia Ave., turn south. The blocks of Andersonville between Broadway and N. Clark St. are lined with hundreds of gracious Victorian homes; most have been lovingly restored in recent years. These blocks kept to themselves while neighboring areas had their post-World War II ups and downs, and if brought here blindfolded, you might think you were in Oak Park.

- After two blocks, turn west on W. Berwyn Ave. and then north on N. Lakewood Ave. Walk two long blocks north (about a quarter of a mile), enjoying the variety of houses on their grassy set-backs (the better for eyeing your neighbors from the front porch), including these highlights: 5313, with a dark lavender and mauve color scheme that boldly sets it apart, as do the unusually tall windows; 5344, a carpenter's gingerbread special that's a painter's dream (if the pay is by the hour); 5426, with an unusual turret and a build date of 1893; 5438, with a flamboyant rising sun on the cornice; and 5448, which somehow got into the punchbowl.

  At W. Catalpa Ave., turn west for two blocks, then south for one block on N. Glenwood Ave. and west for one block on W. Rascher Ave. When you reach N. Clark St., you'll understand the value of the pleasant residential detour that took you away from the urban horror of the Jewel Supermarket parking lot.

- Turn south on Clark St. Andersonville rewards browsers with its plethora of interesting shops, galleries, cafes and bars. A very few highlights, just to give you an idea: Erickson Jewelers, which features a striking façade from the 1940s; Andie's, the best and most characterful of several Middle Eastern restaurants here; Erickson's Deli, the place for lutefisk and less-smelly Swedish specialties like lingonberries; Women and Children First, a fiercely independent bookstore that's a neighborhood treasure; and Presence, a hip women's boutique started by two hippies in 1969. But don't be constrained by these choices; there are dozens more on and off Clark St., for several blocks north and south.

- Cross W. Foster Ave. and you're but 100 feet from our favorite bar. In the 1990s, Michael Roper set about creating his idea of the perfect neighborhood bar, stocked with the beers from the one country in the world with a real beer culture, Belgium, as well as the best microbrews of the Midwest. He succeeded beyond his wildest dreams, and today the Hopleaf is a thriving tavern, with a Belgian cafe (think mussels and frites) and lines often out the door. But it still has no TV, and locals know how to snag a booth near the front bar.

- From N. Clark St., the Red Line El stop at Berwyn is a half-mile walk east, or you can catch the frequent 22 Clark bus.

CONNECTING THE WALKS

You can combine the Foster Beach portion of this walk with Montrose Beach and Walk 26 by walking south along the lake for three-quarters of a mile.

POINTS OF INTEREST

Borders Bookstore 4718 N. Broadway, 773-334-7338

Green Mill 4802 N. Broadway, 773-878-5552

Demera Ethiopian 4801 N. Broadway, 773-334-8787

Annoyance Theater 4830 N. Broadway, 773-561-4665

Thai Grocery 5014 N. Broadway, 773-561-5345

Big Chicks 5024 N. Sheridan Rd., 773-728-5511

Flourish Bakery Cafe 1138 W. Bryn Mawr Ave., 773-271-2253

Kate the Greats 5550 N. Broadway, 773-561-1932

Alchemy Arts 1203 W. Bryn Mawr Ave., 773-769-4970

Erickson Jewelers 5304 N. Clark St., 773-275-2010

Andie's 5253 N. Clark St., 773-784-8616

Erickson's Deli 5250 N. Clark St., 773-561-5634

Women and Children First 5233 N. Clark St., 773-769-9299

Presence 5216 N. Clark St., 773-989-4420

Hopleaf 5148 N. Clark St., 773-334-9851

route summary

1. Start at W. Wilson Ave. and N. Broadway.
2. Head north on N. Broadway.
3. Turn right on W. Argyle St.
4. After three blocks, turn left on N. Sheridan Rd.
5. At W. Winona St., turn right to the lake and cross into Lincoln Park at N. Marine Dr.
6. Follow park paths north and east, crossing under Lake Shore Dr. on W. Foster Ave.
7. Walk north along the lakefront for about half a mile to the W. Bryn Mawr Ave. underpass and head west.
8. Walk west on W. Bryn Mawr Ave. and cross to the west side of N. Broadway.
9. Turn left and walk south on Broadway.
10. Turn right on W. Catalpa Ave. and walk west for one block.
11. At N. Magnolia Ave., turn left.
12. After two blocks, turn right on W. Berwyn Ave. and then right on N. Lakewood Ave.
13. At W. Catalpa Ave., turn left and walk for two blocks.
14. Turn left and go one block south on N. Glenwood Ave.
15. Turn right on W. Rascher Ave.
16. Turn left on N. Clark St.

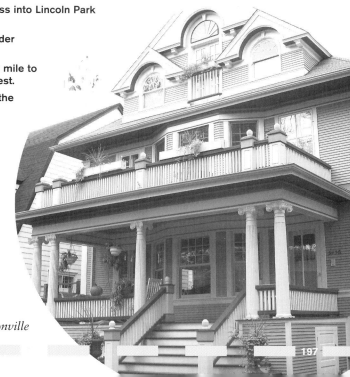

5438 N. Lakewood, Andersonville

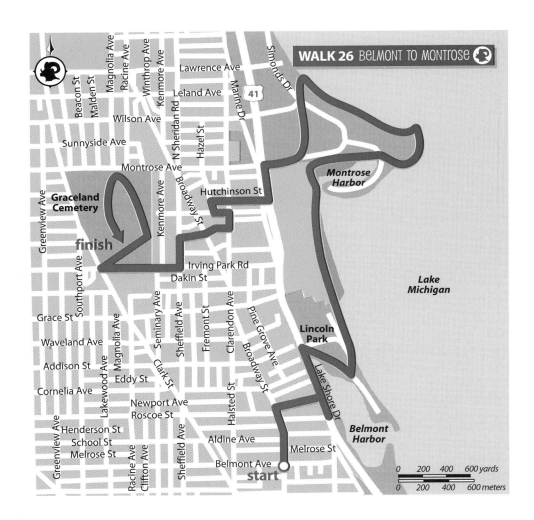

Magnolia Ave
Racine Ave
Winthrop Ave
Kenmore Ave

Lawrence Ave

Leland Ave

Simonds Dr

Beacon St
Malden St

Wilson Ave

Marine Dr

41

N Sheridan Rd

Hazel St

Sunnyside Ave

Montrose Ave

Kenmore Ave

Broadway St

Hutchinson St

Montrose Harbor

Greenview Ave

Graceland Cemetery

finish

Irving Park Rd

Dakin St

Lake Michigan

Grace St

Southport Ave

Seminary Ave

Sheffield Ave

Fremont St

Clarendon Ave

Pine Grove Ave

Broadway St

Lincoln Park

Waveland Ave

Magnolia Ave

Addison St

Lakewood Ave

Clark St

Eddy St

Cornelia Ave

Halsted St

Lake Shore Dr

Newport Ave

Roscoe St

Greenview Ave

Henderson St

School St

Melrose St

Racine Ave

Clifton Ave

Sheffield Ave

Aldine Ave

Melrose St

Belmont Harbor

Belmont Ave

start

0   200   400   600 yards

0   200   400   600 meters

26 BeLMONT TO MONTrose: THe rICH, THe Poor, THe LIVING aND THe DeaD

BOUNDARIES: W. Wilson Ave., Lake Michigan, W. Belmont Ave., N. Clark St.
DISTANCE: 6.6 miles
PUBLIC TRANSIT: 36 Broadway, 77 Belmont, 151 Sheridan busses

Chicago's lakefront becomes more interesting as you go north. Starting at Belmont Harbor, there are twists and turns, paisley-shaped harbors, and crescent-curved beaches. In some parts the shore is far enough from Lake Shore Dr. that traffic noises fade, and on a quiet day you may hear only birds and the lapping of tiny waves on the sand. Lake View is a checkerboard of varied communities; on this walk you'll see neighborhoods popular with the young and partying as well as the filthy rich. And just to remind you that all good things must come to an end, it finishes at the city's last word in final resting places.

- Start your walk at N. Broadway and W. Belmont Ave. This has long been a neighborhood of young professionals enjoying their move to the big city. Cheap apartments abound. The sexual vibe is very mixed; Boystown is a few blocks west, the post-frat and sorority scene on Clark St. not much farther.

- Walk north on Broadway for one block. On Saturdays the playground of the rather attractive 1892 Louis Nettelhorst Public School at N. Melrose St. is the site of the Chicago French Market, a market that differs from the scores of other city-run markets in a few key areas: the awnings look, well, French, you can buy fresh baguettes, there's a guy who bottles his own olive oil, and there are vendors— including one specializing in rubber ducks.

- Across Broadway is the Melrose Restaurant, which features standard diner fare served to customers that might be auditioning for an improv version of *Seinfeld*. Our favorite overheard line: "I could tell he liked me by the way he closed the refrigerator." Okay, get that ring finger ready! In the next block, Unabridged Books is an independent store with gay and lesbian titles, kids' books, a good travel section, and a lot more.

- After a slight kink in Broadway—and no, we don't mean the goings-on at The Closet, a genial bar where the road curves—take a right and go east on W. Hawthorne Pl. In a neighborhood blighted by 4+1's (the notorious early 1960s ugly apartment buildings built by the hundreds so that dozens of units could be crammed onto what had been the plot of a single-family house; one of the reasons so many young folks live around here), this block boasts several standout old mansions. Ones to look for include: 587, an unrestored Craftsman gem with a hammock hanging on the second floor veranda; 580, where sumptuous plantings contrast with sleek Art Deco details; 568, which dates from 1884 and has a splendid wrap-around porch; and 567, now part of the Chicago Day School (a private elementary academy); it has a striking turret spanning three floors.

- At Inner Lake Shore Dr., turn south and walk a little over a block to the pedestrian underpass to the lake. Try not to take a running leap onto the cool blue playground directly in front of the underpass exit. Kid-sized boats are tossed in the "waves" of this rather seductively bouncy ocean. Of course, try to look as if you're determining its suitability for your child.

- Walk north along the water. Belmont Harbor is popular with sailboat owners for the obvious reasons that it's well-sheltered and there's no pesky bridge fouling up the entrance. It boasts both a good yacht club and a sailing school.

- After about 200 yards, there's another scene some may be tempted to join: a fenced beach is one of the city's few areas set aside expressly for dog owners. Fidos and Spots frolic in the water and make new friends and mark turf with abandon. If you venture in, don't go barefoot. (It's also one of the city's great singles spots, for what better way to break the ice than to ask: "Does he do any tricks?")

- Walk north to the tip of the appendix-shaped nub of Belmont Harbor and turn east. Right ahead of you are woods; skirt these to the right for 100 yards and then take the path that follows the fence around the trees toward the lake. At 6½ acres, the Bill Jarvis Migratory Bird Sanctuary is just big enough to feel like a little chunk of Wisconsin. As you follow the fence around, the traffic noise from Lake Shore Dr. fades away. On the west side, a narrow path leads to a raised viewing platform with signs detailing which feathered friends you're likely to see. No points for spotting a dove, which everybody knows is just a pigeon with an agent, but take your time, listen carefully, and you may spot/hear woodpeckers. Crows and swifts are also common. Big money sightings include black-crowned night herons and loons (and we don't mean the guy lurking in the shrubs).

● From the backside of the bird sanctuary, walk to the lake and turn north. The next three-quarters of a mile is surprisingly serene, given that you're a couple minutes' walk from Lake View. On your left is the immaculate green expanse of the par-36 Sydney R. Marovitz Golf Course. It's busy year-round—in winter, fanatical duffers hop the fence and play with colored balls. On your right is an open stretch of Lake Michigan, the waters lapping against the old stone revetments under your feet. A few families try for fish, and should you encounter other walkers, expect a smile that says: "You found this place too, huh?"

● As you come even with the small anchorage at Montrose Harbor, follow the water east past the moorings until the path curves past an open natural area (the path continues south on the harbor's hook-breakwater, but ignore this). This is the Montrose Point Bird Sanctuary, and it's something of a legend with the peeper set, as over 300 species of birds have been spotted amongst the dunes, shrubs, and grasslands. Besides the crew back south at Jarvis, here you can see snowy owls, peregrine falcons, and make truly rare sight-ings, including the bird that gets our vote for superior branding, the Hudsonian godwit.

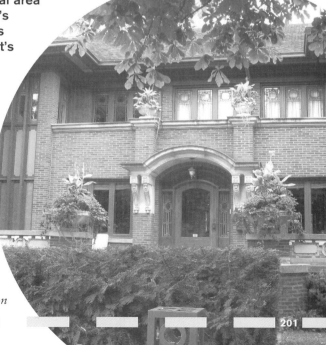

● Walk north along the water to the small patch of dunes at the east end of Montrose Beach. They're a welcome bit of unmanicured sandy

839 W. Hutchinson

goodness, and we wouldn't blame you if you just roll around for a bit. The beach itself gets crowded in summer, and is something of a scene. Follow the shore northwest for about 1,000 yards and you'll come upon a sight that's right out of an Al Gore nightmare: the former boat launch ramps, now high, dry and 100 feet from the water due to falling lake levels. Yikes.

- Head directly south. On weekends the grassy spaces are alive with some of the best amateur soccer league action in the city. Push-cart vendors abound; it's your choice, from tamales to Eskimo pies. Walk up the gentle slope of Cricket Hill (elev: approx. 30 feet) for views in all directions. If you remembered your kite you'll be in good company, otherwise your pleasure will have to be vicarious.

- From the hill, walk down to the path that will take you west through the W. Montrose St. underpass below Lake Shore Dr. On the west side, turn south on N. Marine Dr. and walk to W. Hutchinson St.

- From 1890 to 1920 a stately collection of mansions was built on the two blocks west of here. Many of the later ones are Prairie-style, and show the design revolution this represented when compared to the Queen Anne, Romanesque, and other styles on the street. The highlights are many; here are a few: 750, whose broad curved windows overlook a huge side yard behind Roman-brick walls; 803, where the porte cochere is worthy of a hotel—or a funeral home; 817, the stately order of Prairie style marches across the façade; 826, deceptively simple at first, with more of its calculated details emerging the longer you look; 839, where the brass sign on the gate says: THIS ANIMAL IS DANGEROUS. PLEASE DON'T FEED OR DISTURB. Is it an animal? A resident? Weird Uncle Homer in the attic? Finally, there's 840, a vision out of Grimm's Fairy Tales.

- At the west end of Hutchinson, turn sharply south on N. Hazel St., jog slightly east when you hit W. Buena Ave., then go south on N. Clarendon Ave. two short blocks to W. Belle Plaine Ave. On the northeast corner, Dollop Coffee Co. is a neighborhood fave for its fine coffees, snacks, tables outside, free wi-fi and lack of faux Italian pretension. If you want a large, you say "large."

- Follow the gentle S-curve of W. Belle Plaine Ave. for two blocks across N. Broadway to N. Sheridan Rd. Turn south. This area was a gracious middle-class neighborhood 100 years ago. For a multitude of reasons it hit the skids in the 1970s, and now has clawed its way back.

- At W. Irving Park Rd., take a right and walk under the El tracks and on for another quarter of a mile. To your south is Wunder's Cemetery, a weedy place that doesn't live up to its name. On your north, however, is Chicago's cemetery to the stars. When you reach N. Clark St., make a sharp turn and enter Graceland Cemetery. Ignoring for a minute the urge to airily utter, "A lot of people are dying to get in here," pause and get a sense of where you are. Established in 1860, Graceland's 121 acres became *the* place for eternal rest. A virtual Who's Who of Chicagoans are here, often interred in tombs designed by leading architects, who when they died, joined their clients at Graceland. Stop by the discreet little office and pick up the free maps or, better, buy the first-rate guidebook. The delightful staff will even help you plan your tour, which can easily run a mile or more. Noteworthy residents include: liquor-dealer and city founder John Kinzie; capitalist George Pullman (who, fearing that some of the legions of workers he had stiffed would come desecrating, had his tomb armor-plated); Potter and Bertha Palmer, the original power-couple with a nice waterside retreat; Daniel "make no little plans" Burnham, who is on a little shady island in the lake; architect Louis Sullivan, who died nearly broke and who has a simple headstone near the grand monuments he designed for others in better times; and Marshall Field, whose tomb is topped by a statue of a woman looking so desolate that she might be reacting to the takeover of his namesake store by Macy's 100 years after his death.

- The 22 Clark and 80 Irving Park busses run frequently past Graceland's entrance.

CONNECTING THE WALKS

You can combine the lakefront portion of this walk with Walk 25 that covers Foster Beach by walking three-quarters of a mile north to Montrose Beach. From Belmont Harbor, walk south three-quarters of a mile to Diversey Harbor and join Walk 22.

POINTS OF INTEREST

Melrose Restaurant 3233 N. Broadway, 773-327-2060

Unabridged Books 3251 N. Broadway, 773-883-9119

The Closet 3333 N. Broadway, 773-477-8533

Dollop Coffee Co. 4181 N. Clarendon St., 773-755-1955

Graceland Cemetery 4001 N. Clark St., 773-525-1105

ROUTE SUMMARY

1. Start your walk at N. Broadway and W. Belmont Ave.
2. Walk north on Broadway.
3. Turn right on W. Hawthorne Pl.
4. At Inner Lake Shore Dr., turn right and walk a little over a block to the pedestrian underpass to the lake.
5. Walk north along the water at Belmont Harbor.
6. Walk north to the tip of Belmont Harbor and turn east. Right ahead of you are woods; skirt these to the right for 100 yards and then take the path that follows the fence around the trees toward the lake.
7. Walk to the lake and turn north.
8. At Montrose Harbor, follow the water east past the moorings until the path curves past an open natural area (ignore the path going south onto the breakwater).
9. Walk north along the water to the small patch of dunes at the east end of Montrose Beach.
10. Follow the shore northwest for about 1,000 yards.
11. Head directly south and walk up Cricket Hill.

12. From the hill, walk down to the path west through the W. Montrose St. underpass below Lake Shore Dr. On the west side, turn left on N. Marine Dr. and walk to W. Hutchinson St. Turn right.

13. At the west end of Hutchinson, turn sharply left on N. Hazel St., jog slightly east when you hit W. Buena Ave., then turn right and go south on N. Clarendon Ave. two short blocks to W. Belle Plaine Ave.

14. Follow W. Belle Plaine Ave. for two blocks across N. Broadway to N. Sheridan Rd. Turn left.

15. At W. Irving Park Rd., turn right on N. Clark St.

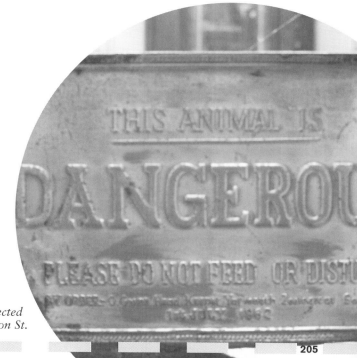

Privilege has always been protected
on W. Hutchinson St.

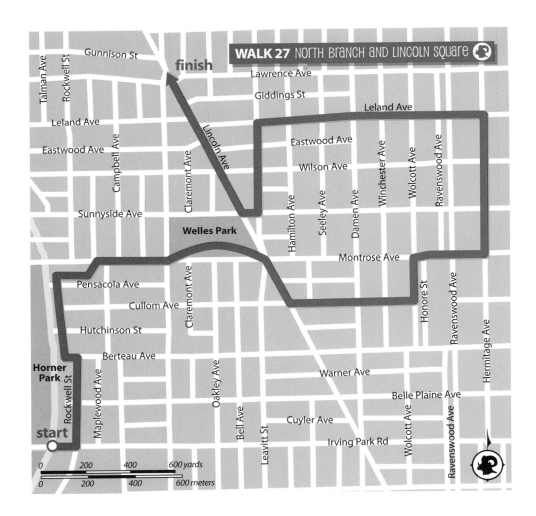

finish

Gunnison St

Talman Ave

Rockwell St

Lawrence Ave

Giddings St

Leland Ave

Leland Ave

Eastwood Ave

Eastwood Ave

Campbell Ave

Wilson Ave

Winchester Ave

Wolcott Ave

Ravenswood Ave

Lincoln Ave

Sunnyside Ave

Claremont Ave

Welles Park

Hamilton Ave

Seeley Ave

Damen Ave

Montrose Ave

Ravenswood Ave

Pensacola Ave

Cullom Ave

Claremont Ave

Honore St

Hutchinson St

Berteau Ave

Horner Park

Rockwell St

Maplewood Ave

Warner Ave

Oakley Ave

Belle Plaine Ave

Wolcott Ave

Ravenswood Ave

Hermitage Ave

start

Bell Ave

Leavitt St

Cuyler Ave

Irving Park Rd

0   200   400   600 yards
0   200   400   600 meters

27 NOrTH Branch and LINCOLN Square: OLD TradiTIONs, New WeaLTH

BOUNDARIES: **W. Lawrence Ave., N. Hermitage Ave., W. Irving Park Rd., Chicago River North Branch**
DISTANCE: **3.7 miles**
PUBLIC TRANSIT: **80 Irving Park bus to N. Rockwell St.**

Just as the Chicago River has been rediscovered as an amenity downtown, so it has on the North Side, where massive efforts have cleaned it up enough that it's popular with fish, birds, and people again. A unique community-built riverwalk gives a good glimpse of what's here. The adjoining community of Lincoln Square is officially "hot" right now, with no short-age of fine places to eat, drink, and shop. There's little doubt that its founders more than 100 years ago would be very pleased with its current state—and they'd no doubt appreciate the healthy growth in real estate prices.

- Start your walk on the N. Irving Park Rd. Bridge over the North Branch of the Chicago River. Look north at a little bit of the country in the city. Ducks paddle across the sur-face, small boats line the banks, and low-hanging trees blur the definition between water and land. For a better view, walk east slightly and then two blocks north on N. Rockwell St. This short stretch perfectly encapsulates the modern story of the North Branch: at first there are some light industrial buildings, but then you find that one of the places that once made widgets has been turned into a high-end dog hotel, where pampered pooches receive better treatment than the workers here ever did. As you near W. Berteau Ave., the scene changes to a row of upscale houses, sold to people who see the river as an amenity, rather than a blight.

- Turn west and walk to the bank above the water. Starting here and running for a quarter of a mile north is a community-built and maintained riverwalk. For well more than a decade, neighbors here have banded together to restore the natural edge of the riverbank, plant and propagate native plants, and make the Chicago River acces-sible to anyone.

- Turn north along the path, noting the low fences woven from twigs and branches fallen from the trees above. For decades, the very idea of expending sweat to bring people closer to the river would have been greeted by derisive hoots. Although much attention was focused on the South Branch and its industrial squalor at places like Bubbly Creek, the North Branch wasn't treated much better. It was often little more than a relief valve for sewage and other wastes. Now after billions of dollars spent on water treatment, flood control, and bribes, the water quality has reached the point where more than 70 species of fish can be found in its admittedly olive-drab waters.

- Stroll the meandering path; note that many people have canoes and kayaks tied up to the bank. Just a few years ago, a plunge into the Chicago River would have sparked the lighting of votive candles; now your fate would probably be limited to the jab of a tetanus shot. (Although signs warning of contact with the water from the Metropolitan Water Reclamation District are a definite buzz kill.) The path dips up and down along the bank, and fenced yards and dead-end streets help the tranquility. At the end of W. Cullom St., there's a nice, naturalistic tiered seating area. Signs written by the neighbors detail the large number of birds, like coots, swans, kingfishers, and grebes that can be spotted; one gives nice insight into how this whole area was marshy prairie less than 300 years ago.

- As you near the W. Montrose Ave. Bridge, the path ends. Cut east along the alley behind the old apartment buildings, and after about 100 yards there's a parking lot. Cut across this to Montrose Ave. and walk east.

- After your short jaunt through nature, you may be ready for sustenance. There's no better way to return to urban life than at Lutz Cafe and Pastry Shop, where butter-cream is a staple, not a treat. Slow the blood racing through your arteries with one of the oozing tarts or lavish cakes displayed in the cases. Nothing's changed here in 50 years; posters of Tony Bennett keep you company in the bathrooms.

- Crossing N. Western Ave., forsake the Montrose sidewalk for the Welles Park paths. Covering just over 15 acres, the park is a real anchor for the community. Lap-swimmers fill the indoor pool year-round, local musicians perform at the elaborate sound-equipped gazebo in summer, and fall kid's football leagues are just some of the teams competing on the sod.

- Turn south on N. Lincoln Ave. and walk into the pedantically named North Center neighborhood. Until boosters rebrand the place something like Northwest Lincoln Park Prairie, the bland name will unnecessarily temper expectations for what's a rather tidy and delightful place (okay, maybe the name is spot on). The diagonal of Lincoln Ave. is lined with some tasty casual eateries. A dramatic second-floor bay window calls attention to Chalkboard, which has won raves for its changing menu of seasonal American food. Just south, on the northeast corner with W. Pensacola Ave., Jury's Food and Drink is an upscale pub with much-loved burgers and plenty of tipples by the glass.

- Just south of the intersection with W. Cullom Ave., the cries of anguish or joy you hear may be coming from fans in the sports bars that bookend Lincoln. To get so close to the action you can almost smell it, look for the tiny Stadium Seat Store on the east side of the street. For $300 you can have a Wrigley Field seat where generations of Cubs fans sat through decades of disappointment. Don't dwell on the thousands of butts that rested here during an afternoon of beer-swilling, and chili- and sauerkraut-slathered hot-dog pounding.

- Dart back up to Cullom and walk east about a third of a mile to N. Wolcott Ave., and then north one block to W. Montrose Ave. Walk west, first crossing under the El and then the Metra tracks, which carry trains full of swells to the upscale suburbs on the North Shore. The tracks are lined with small warehouses and commercial buildings dating from the 1910s when light industries like postcard printers and pigment grinders provided jobs for the Germans and Swedes who filled the modest two- and three-flats.

Carl Sandburg wrote here, 4646 N. Hermitage Ave.

- Walk north on N. Hermitage Ave. through the heart of Ravenswood. These blocks nicely reflect the neighborhood's current popularity. The mix of single and multi-family homes are mostly renovated. In October, Chicago's ever-growing obsession with outdoor Halloween decorations means that every block has trees filled with ghouls, lawns lined with tombstones, and pumpkins grinning from porch to porch.

- On the southwest corner with W. Wilson Ave., the peeling paint and sagging eaves do little to honor All Saints Episcopal Church. When built in 1891, it sat alone in Norman Rockwell-esque splendor on an open prairie of farms and wildflowers.

- Continue north on Hermitage. Note the eclectic mansion at 4605, one of the first built after the church. Mid-block, look for the three-flat at 4646. Carl Sandburg moved here in 1912 and worked as a newspaper reporter and editor. But after hours he labored at the second-floor flat here writing poetry, including the iconic *Chicago* ("Hog-butcher, tool-maker, stacker of wheat, player with railroads, and freight-handler to the nation.") In 1926 he wrote a biography of Abraham Lincoln, which brought him both acclaim and money, allowing him to move to a succession of larger homes in the country.

- At the end of the block, turn west on W. Leland Ave., walk seven blocks west to N. Leavitt St., and turn south. The visual harmony of these blocks is only occasionally interrupted by recent grandiose McMansions. Shame.

- Walk south until you see the bulk of the Sulzer Regional Library, the perfect intellectual companion to previously mentioned Welles Park across the street. Turn west briefly and then north on N. Lincoln Ave. On the west side of the street, look for the 1930s municipal building. The owl on the façade hints that this was the former home for the library. In a brilliant bit of reuse, it's now home to the Old Town School of Folk Music, an institution started in the then-Bohemian neighborhood to the south. In 1998 it opened these vast new quarters, which serve over 6,000 students a week. Classes include Clawhammer Banjo 1 and Ukulele Ensemble. The school has preserved two splendid WPA murals from the children's reading room of the old library.

- On the east side of the street across W. Wilson Ave., you will not miss the last commissions of the great architect Louis Sullivan. By 1922, alcoholism and irascibility had reduced the architect of the Auditorium Building to working as a designer for a terra-cotta company (given what he did with the material, they owed him). The façade on the former Krause Music Store is a masterpiece in miniature. The current occupant, a visual communications firm owned by Peter and Pooja Vukosavich, has completed an award-winning restoration, and added a serene garden you can glimpse out back.

- Cross under the El tracks. As this part of Chicago has been revitalized in recent years, ridership on the Brown Line above has soared. Lincoln Ave. bends off to the west as part of an old urban renewal scheme. There's limited traffic north in the heart of the old Lincoln Square commercial district. Long a hub for North Side German-Americans, you can still smell the sausage today at places like the old-school Huettenbar (slogan: "Meet your next best friend here.") and the Chicago Brauhaus. There's a good range of businesses that aren't simply trading on German schtick, including Merz Apothecary, which makes much of being a living museum of homeopathic cures, and the Book Cellar, a modern indie bookseller with a good cafe.

- Just across busy W. Lawrence Ave., there's a statue of Abraham Lincoln that shows the square's honoree in his younger days. The inscription is his 1856 quote: "Free society is not, and shall not be, a failure." Where's Abe when we need him? (At least you have the freedom to buy fresh corn at the farmers market here on Tuesdays.)

- The modern Brown Line El stop at Western makes a handy exit from the neighborhood.

CONNECTING THE WALKS

Catch the 81 Lawrence bus heading east and link up with Walk 25.

POINTS OF INTEREST

Lutz Cafe and Pastry Shop 2458 W. Montrose Ave., 773-478-7785

Chalkboard 4343 N. Lincoln Ave., 773-477-7144

Jury's Food and Drink 4337 N. Lincoln Ave., 773-935-2255

Stadium Seat Store 4251 N. Lincoln Ave., 773-404-7975

Old Town School of Folk Music www.oldtownschool.org, 4544 N. Lincoln Ave., 773-751-3398

Huettenbar 4721 N. Lincoln Ave., 773-561-2507

Chicago Brauhaus 4732 N. Lincoln Ave., 773-784-4444

Merz Apothecary 4716 N. Lincoln Ave., 773-989-0900

Book Cellar 4736 N. Lincoln Ave., 773-293-2665

ROUTE SUMMARY

1. Start on the N. Irving Park Rd. Bridge over the North Branch of the Chicago River.
2. Walk east slightly and then turn left and go two blocks north on N. Rockwell St.
3. Turn left and walk to the bank above the water.
4. Turn right along the path.
5. As you near the W. Montrose Ave. Bridge, the path ends. Cut east along the alley behind the old apartment buildings and after about 100 yards, cut across a parking lot to Montrose Ave. and walk east.
6. Crossing N. Western Ave., walk east through Welles Park.
7. Turn right on N. Lincoln Ave.
8. Turn left on W. Cullom Ave. and walk about a third of a mile to N. Wolcott Ave.

9.   Turn left and walk one block to W. Montrose Ave.

10. Turn right and go east, first crossing under the El and then the Metra tracks.

11. Turn left on N. Hermitage Ave.

12. Turn left on W. Leland Ave. and walk seven blocks.

13. Turn left and walk four blocks on N. Leavitt St.

14. Turn west briefly where Leavitt meets N. Lincoln Ave. and then go north.

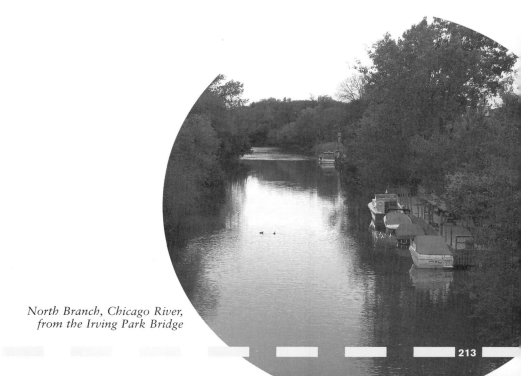

*North Branch, Chicago River,
from the Irving Park Bridge*

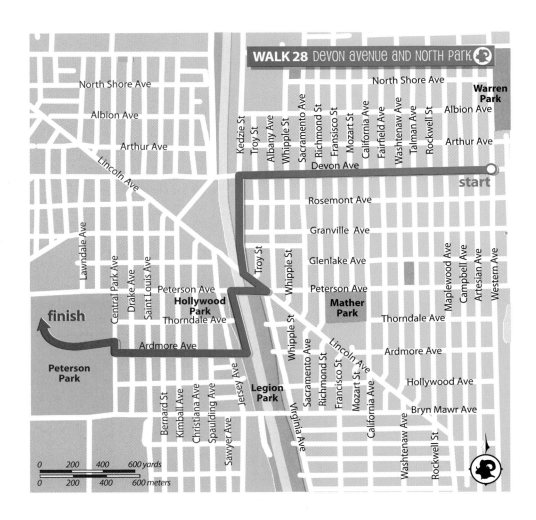

North Shore Ave

North Shore Ave

Warren Park

Albion Ave

Albion Ave

Arthur Ave

Arthur Ave

Lincoln Ave

Kedzie St

Troy St

Albany Ave

Whipple St

Sacramento Ave

Richmond St

Fransisco St

Mozart St

California Ave

Fairfield Ave

Washtenaw Ave

Talman Ave

Rockwell St

Devon Ave

start

Rosemont Ave

Lawndale Ave

Central Park Ave

Drake Ave

Saint Louis Ave

Troy St

Whipple St

Granville Ave

Glenlake Ave

Peterson Ave

Maplewood Ave

Campbell Ave

Artesian Ave

Western Ave

finish

Peterson Ave

Hollywood Park

Thorndale Ave

Mather Park

Thorndale Ave

Ardmore Ave

Whipple St

Lincoln Ave

Ardmore Ave

Peterson Park

Bernard St

Kimball Ave

Christiana Ave

Spaulding Ave

Sawyer Ave

Jersey Ave

Legion Park

Sacramento Ave

Richmond St

Francisco St

Mozart St

Virginia Ave

California Ave

Hollywood Ave

Bryn Mawr Ave

Washtenaw Ave

Rockwell St

0   200   400   600 yards

0   200   400   600 meters

28 Devon Avenue and North Park: Around the World in an Afternoon

BOUNDARIES: **W. Devon Ave., N. Western Ave., W. Bryn Mawr Ave., N. Pulaski Rd.**
DISTANCE: **2¾ miles**
PUBLIC TRANSIT: **49B North Western and 155 Devon busses**

Chicago has always been well-known for its multitude of ethnic communities. Taking a trip abroad just by hopping the El is one of the city's great pleasures. What seems like half the city's ethnic groups can be found in West Ridge, a neighborhood on the far North Side that is crossed by W. Devon Ave. Along this endlessly fascinating street you can cross the Middle East and South Asia in less than a mile. One minute you're munching an Indian chickpea snack, the next you're enjoying lox. In sharp contrast, less than a mile away, the city's one nature center can transport you to a rural, woodsy retreat that seems almost as far away. And you can do it all in an afternoon.

● Begin your walk at N. Western Ave. and W. Devon Ave. The stretch of Western to the south has the honorary name "King Sargon Blvd." in honor of the ancient ruler of much of Mesopotamia. It's the first of a virtual Babel of honorary names that seem to change with every block. Walk west, through a fairly cluttered bit of Devon, with shops selling cheap calls to the Eastern Hemisphere, electronics joints peddling brands never before seen, cut-rate variety stores, and more.

● Past N. Campbell Ave. look for Arya Bhavan, one of the more notable among many Indian restaurants along Devon. The pink napkins fanned out across the tables provide a dash of color to go with excellent Northern Indian vegetarian cuisine. Chicago's Indian population is growing fast, and surpassed 60,000 in 2000. Pop into any of the surrounding sari shops for a polychromatic explosion of textiles.

● At the next corner, N. Maplewood Ave., turn south for 50 feet off Devon and look for the little storefront of the Mughal Bakery on the west side. The ovens are always on and a constant stream of Pakistani breads and cookies issues forth. Many are bought by waiting customers before they even touch a counter. Look cheery and you're likely to be handed a treat, which you can enjoy at one of the many benches near this and other street corners (although you may have entrenched competition from hordes of old men who gather on the benches for spirited debates and gossip). Estimates of the Pakistani population in Chicago vary, but 40,000 is a median number.

- Back on Devon, you're within a few feet of India Book House, where you can get a DVD of the latest Bollywood sensation. Almost next door (thousands of saris intervene) is Sukhadia's, an Indian bakery and sweet shop. After some Mughal cookies, a mango shake at this purple palace goes down a treat.

- West of N. Rockwell St., several markets sell a vast range of foodstuffs you won't find at your local Jewel. Fresh Farms International Market on Devon stocks something for almost everyone, and feels like a huge bazaar. Goods range from Sinquas (giant okras) to long, tuberous Chinese eggplant. Buy a fresh coconut and they'll whack off the top, insert a straw, and give you biodegradable refreshment.

- Past Talman Ave., Kamdar Plaza sells *khandvia*, a South Asian treat that's sort of like a steamed crepe, but made with chickpea (garbanzo bean) flour and yoghurt, then garnished with cilantro, coconut, chilies, and mustard seeds, with tamarind chutney on the side. That it's delicious is something Indians and Pakistanis both agree on.

- And amidst this United Nations of cultures, how could a few blocks go by without an Irish bar? Casey's Corner (at N. Fairfield Ave.) is pure dive and has proudly been so for over 80 years.

- As you near N. California Ave., the scene begins shifting to the Middle East. A classic well-lit bookshop, Iqra Book Center has a large selection of Islamic titles, many under their own imprint. There are large children's and language sections. Nearby, you'll see several meat markets selling "Zabiha meat," a method of slaughtering meat that's more strict in its procedures than Halal, the certification required by Muslims. These stores draw customers from across the Midwest. Many of Chicago's Middle Eastern restaurants are run by Lebanese who first came to Chicago to work as artisans for the 1893 Columbian Exposition.

- Passing California (that's the street, this isn't that wild of a tour), it's time to take a trip north to the shores of the Black Sea. (And in honor of this, you'll want to use the north side of the street, as the south side is a lengthy desert of a CVS Pharmacy and parking lot.) Argo Georgian Bakery has one of Chicago's only traditional dome-shaped ovens, which has no logo on it but should say: "Take that, Kitchen Aid. Up Yours Wolf," because of the amazing goods cooked within. There are flaky-as-a-cheerleader fresh raspberry tarts, filling lavash (round flatbread) and addictive khachapuri (a pastry of many cheeses). Chicago's small Georgian community got its start after the collapse of the Soviet Union opened the doors to emigration.

- At the corner of N. Mozart St., note that rather than honor a specific individual to represent an ethnic group, the city in its unstinting efforts to leave no constituent unappeased has given the south block the honorary title of "Croatia Drive."

- Past Mozart, it's Russian at Three Sisters, an aromatic deli named for the Chekhov (as in Anton the writer, not Pavel the photon-torpedo-shooter) play about the decay of the upper classes and the lure of the bright lights of Moscow. Although the lights in this spotless store are bright, the allure here is smoked fish, all manner of pickled goods, prepared dishes like blintzes, and cured meats. Go on, ask the uniformed matrons behind the counter if they're sisters.

- About a block and half farther on is a place where the language is universal: since 1951 the Music House has been offering classes in instruments from violins to woodwind to brass. They have programs throughout the Chicago schools.

Park in North Park Village

● Much of Devon Ave. on this walk was Jewish through the 1960s. Since then, many of the original residents have moved on to various suburbs, and many other ethnic groups have moved in. However, there's still a close-knit Jewish community west of N. Francisco St., many with the distinct appearance of Hasidic Jews. One of the hubs is Good Morgan, a deli that has fun with the owner's name (Aaron Morgan). Whitefish in every form imaginable (smoked, fried, grilled, etc.) is sold to go or for consumption at the crowded tables in the blue- and white-tiled dining area. If the food doesn't put a smile on your face, the jaunty fish on the sign out front will. Farther west, past N. Sacramento Ave., the prim campus on the south side of Devon is Hanna Sacks Bais Yaakov High School.

● From N. Whipple St. west there are several orthodox synagogues and a decreasing number of businesses. The street takes on a typically post-war character, which means that it's not very interesting. Fortunately, when you reach N. Kedzie Ave. you turn south. Walk past the apartments on the west and the 1950s bungalows on the east until a grassy area appears on the right. Edge your way off Kedzie and walk south along the trees on the bank of the North Branch of the Chicago River. After about 300 yards you'll come to an impressive concrete sidewalk that leads south to a passage under N. Lincoln Ave. If you think it looks like a bike trail you're right. Now look across the river and you'll see a similar path going north past a new senior citizens complex. If you think the two should be linked by a bridge, you'd be right again. However, although the bridge has been funded, it's been blocked by the local alderman out of pure churlishness. One of the senior members of the City Council, Bernard Stone, has no truck with bicyclists. That a recent electoral opponent was a well-known local cyclist certainly didn't help.

● Bridge or no bridge, use the new path to first cross under Lincoln Ave. and then W. Peterson Ave. Now curl back around counter-clockwise and cross the river on Peterson (with the cursing cyclists). On the west side, immediately drop down onto a path that follows the river south. Follow this bucolic—and quiet—greenway for a quarter of a mile and then walk west on W. Ardmore Ave. This is solid middle-class Chicago. A tidy neighborhood of post-war homes that have never been fashionable or unfashionable. Chinese lions flanking some doors, as well as synagogues, reveal the area's ethnic diversity.

- Where Ardmore dead-ends at N. Central Park Ave., take the path through the fence into the large park-like area. This is North Park Village, the center of the surrounding namesake neighborhood, and until 1974 the Municipal Tuberculosis Sanitarium. Today this large and rural-feeling campus has senior apartments, a park, and your destination: the one large nature preserve in the city proper.

- Walk generally west, diverting slightly north to pass by the baseball diamonds of Petersen Park (a more interesting route than the access road). About 250 yards after the park, you'll see a large parking area and north of there a small building housing a nature center. This is the entrance to North Park Village Nature Center, a 46-acre preserve that beautifully recreates a wooded and marshy prairie—just what you would have found across the area 300 years ago. There's little need to linger over the basic displays in the nature center; rather, get out and enjoy the half mile of trails through a landscape rich with wildflowers, lily ponds and a huge variety of trees. Keep a lookout for squirrels, raccoons, deer, chipmunks, turtles, rabbits, and whole bunch of other critters that would populate an entire Disney cartoon. Large birds include two kinds of owls, hawks, and herons. The staff stages special programs through the year and seasonal events such as the spring maple sap-tapping weekend.

- Leaving North Park Village is somewhat easier than returning to civilization from the country. From the nature center, walk west for a quarter of a mile to N. Pulaski Rd. Here you can catch a 53 Pulaski bus south to the Blue Line El stop at Irving Park Rd.

POINTS OF INTEREST

Arya Bhavan 2508 W. Devon Ave., 773-274-5800

Mughal Bakery 6348 N. Maplewood Ave., 773-761-9660

India Book House 2551 W. Devon Ave., 866-656-5999

Sukhadia's 2559 W. Devon Ave., 773-338-5400

Fresh Farms International Market 2626 W. Devon Ave., 773-764-5757

Kamdar Plaza 2646 W. Devon Ave., 773-338-8100

Casey's Corner 2733 W. Devon Ave.

Iqra Book Center 2749 W. Devon Ave., 773-274-2665

Argo Georgian Bakery 2812 W. Devon Ave., 773-764-6322

Three Sisters 2854 W. Devon Ave., 773-465-6695

Music House 2925 W. Devon Ave., 773-262-7309

Good Morgan 2948 W. Devon Ave., 773-764-8115

North Park Village Nature Center 5801 N. Pulaski Rd., 312-744-5472

route summary

1. Begin at N. Western Ave. and W. Devon Ave.
2. Walk west on W. Devon Ave.
3. Turn left on N. Kedzie Ave.
4. Use the new path to first cross under Lincoln Ave. and then W. Peterson Ave.
5. Curl back around counter-clockwise and cross the river on Peterson.
6. On the west side, drop down onto a path that follows the river south.
7. Walk west on W. Ardmore Ave.
8. Take the path through the fence into the large park-like area of North Park Village.
9. Walk west, diverting slightly north to pass by the baseball diamonds of Petersen Park. About 250 yards after the park, you'll see a large parking area and north of there a nature center.

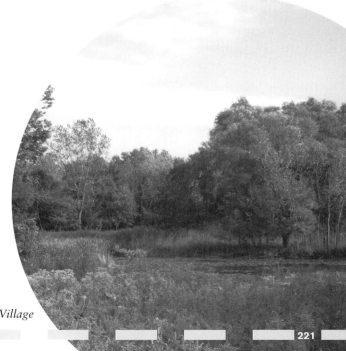

Another view of the park in North Park Village

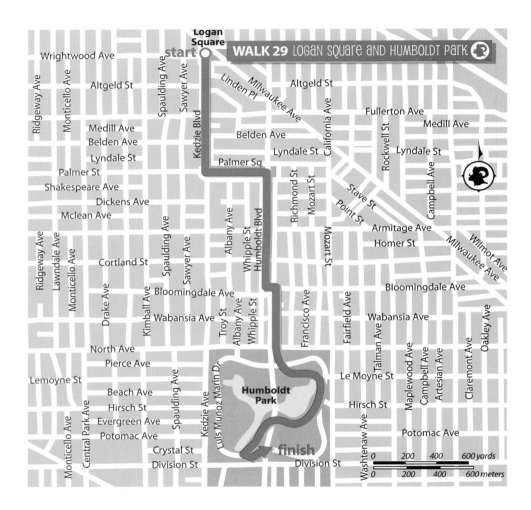

Logan
Square

start

Wrightwood Ave

Ridgeway Ave

Monticello Ave

Altgeld St

Spaulding Ave

Sawyer Ave

Kedzie Blvd

Linden Pl

Milwaukee Ave

Altgeld St

California Ave

Fullerton Ave

Rockwell St

Medill Ave

Medill Ave

Belden Ave

Belden Ave

Lyndale St

Lyndale St

Lyndale St

Palmer St

Palmer Sq

Campbell Ave

Shakespeare Ave

Dickens Ave

Richmond St

Mozart St

Stave St

Point St

Armitage Ave

Mclean Ave

Homer St

Milwaukee Ave

Wilmot Ave

Ridgeway Ave

Lawndale Ave

Monticello Ave

Spaulding Ave

Sawyer Ave

Albany Ave

Whipple St

Humboldt Blvd

Mozart St

Cortland St

Drake Ave

Kimball Ave

Bloomingdale Ave

Bloomingdale Ave

Francisco Ave

Fairfield Ave

Oakley Ave

Claremont Ave

Wabansia Ave

Troy St

Albany Ave

Whipple St

Wabansia Ave

Talman Ave

Maplewood Ave

Campbell Ave

Artesian Ave

North Ave

Pierce Ave

Le Moyne St

Lemoyne St

Spaulding Ave

Kedzie Ave

Luis Munoz Martin Dr

**Humboldt
Park**

Hirsch St

Beach Ave

Hirsch St

Washtenaw Ave

Monticello Ave

Central Park Ave

Evergreen Ave

Potomac Ave

Potomac Ave

Crystal St

finish

Division St

Division St

Division St

| 0 | 200 | 400 | 600 yards |
| 0 | 200 | 400 | 600 meters |

29 LOGaN SQuare aND HUMBOLDT ParK: SuNrise BOuLeVarDs

BOUNDARIES: Logan Square, N. California St., W. Division St., Kedzie Blvd.
DISTANCE: 3¼ miles
PUBLIC TRANSIT: Blue Line El to Logan Square

The best thing about including a walk from Logan Square to Humboldt Park is simply including it. These two areas were much knocked about from the 1930s on as constantly changing demographics and waves of poor immigrants overwhelmed the community's ability to be self-sustaining. Once jewels in the "ring of pearls" that was the Boulevard System (see below), the communities hit the skids. Now things are changing. Logan Square has gentrified, and once-grand rows of houses are grand again; Humboldt Park is following, especially as the Park District is finally giving the namesake park the care and attention it deserves. But these changes are wrenching; the very communities using the Humboldt Park neighborhood as the first stop on the way to a better life are resisting the economic forces pushing them out.

- Start your walk at the *Illinois Centennial Monument* on Logan Square. In the midst of the chaotic maze of converging traffic, the neighborhood's main feature is a pleasant urban respite, if you live long enough to get out to it. The 1918 sculpture celebrating the state's admission to the Union is easily the most dramatic feature in a traffic circle anywhere in the city. An eagle preparing to fly sits atop a 68-foot Doric column made from pink marble, which in turn is on a base with reliefs highlighting the usual suspects (farmers, Native Americans, laborers, etc.) from the state's first 100 years. Sadly, the carvings don't include graft-seeking politicians. The monument itself is on a slight knoll that many use for sun-bathing in summer and viewing the Gothic Norwegian Lutheran Church to the northwest on N. Kedzie Ave. It still has some services in Norwegian—the ethnic group that predominated here before the war.

- Logan Square is a hub in Chicago's Boulevard System of landscaped parkways. Logan Blvd. runs east and is the starting point for Walk 30. This walk goes south on Kedzie Blvd.

Arrayed around the square are several good places to eat. On the southeast corner of Kedzie and N. Milwaukee Ave. are two of note. Johnny's Grill right on the corner has a sign that says THIS ISN'T BURGER KING. YOU DO IT MY WAY. A classic attitude to go with classic diner food. Just outside are two exchange boxes with free books and VHS tapes. The pillars are the area's best bulletin board. The scene couldn't be any more different just south at Lula's Cafe, where even your glass of water comes with a side of hip. The seasonal organic menu reflects what's fresh and is heavy on herbs and bright flavors. But note that such joys have a price: waits of up to two hours on pretty weekends for a sidewalk table.

- Walk south on Kedzie Blvd. This street is typical of Chicago boulevards: a wide middle avenue for through traffic bordered by landscaped medians, with another street on each side for local traffic and parking in front of houses. People building the best houses were drawn to these elegant venues, and Kedzie Blvd. is no exception. Its row of impressive houses stretching south a half mile to Palmer Square is mostly intact. The best ones are on the west side, so make your way across.

- Just north of W. Fullerton Ave. at 2410, the William Nowaczewski House is over-the-top even by the street's standards. Built in 1897, it embodies just about every medieval fantasy short of a pot of boiling oil waiting to be poured out of the turret. Then again, do you want to be the one to find out the truth?

- At W. Fullerton Ave. walk west one block. As Logan Square has gentrified, all manner of trendy places have opened on and off the avenues. Two spots here show that it's possible to be both popular and preserve tradition at the same time. Cigar-sized El Rinconcito Cubano has old photos of pre-Castro Havana and even older men from pre-Castro Cuba to prove that it's no newcomer. The food is amazingly good: garlic infuses a classic line-up of beef, pork and other meaty dishes. One block farther west, look for the lavish terra-cotta building at the southwest corner with S. Spaulding Ave. It's the local outpost for Adidam, a religion founded by Adi Da Samraj (a.k.a. Bubba Free John et al.), who has advocated a faith that mixes Eastern spiritual notions with a pastiche of feel-good frolics.

- Return to Kedzie Blvd. and continue south. The variety of houses continues to lean camp (with a few unwelcome modern duds). Among those worth highlighting are

2312, with its overlay of Prairie-school order, and 2224, which sports an oddball face amidst its Art Nouveau details.

- Kedzie Blvd. runs into Palmer Square (more of an oval, really), easily the most gentrified portion of the walk. Your biggest fear here will be getting run down by a Crate & Barrel delivery truck. The seven-acre central park is uncleaved by a middle avenue of traffic. Instead, it's surrounded by racetrack-shaped W. Palmer Street, which links Kedzie Blvd. with Humboldt Blvd. Walk its quarter-mile length east, while enjoying the mix of 1890s homes lining the edges. Little is unrestored here, and the homes generally go for seven figures. Meanwhile money has been secured to install various amenities like a soft-surface jogging track. Hmmm . . . no wonder the poor folks are pissed.

- At the east end of Palmer Square, turn south on Humboldt Blvd. The southwest corner once held the grand mansion of Ignaz Schwinn, now gone like his bicycle company. (The family lost the brand to bankruptcy in 1994 after they dismissed mountain bikes as a passing fancy. Oops.)

- Humboldt Blvd. runs south to its namesake park for three-quarters of a mile. It bears more scars of the decades than Kedzie Blvd. In many places the trees are quite young, having replaced old elms that were cut down years ago. There's a mixture of large homes, apartments, and newer, cheaper places built as fill-ins during the 1970s. Still, don't think you're safe from that Crate & Barrel truck. Especially on the east side of the street and the blocks beyond, the evil G-word—gentrification— is much in play.

Illinois Centennial Monument, *Logan Square*

- Much of the namesake neighborhood of the park lies to the west. It has always been a place where people landed when they first reached Chicago; Germans, Swedes, Jews, Italians, Poles, in that order through the 1950s. Then as immigration from Puerto Rico picked up in the 1960s, Humboldt Park was again waiting—if not with a warm welcome, at least with a cheap bed. Now, however, gentrification spreading west from Bucktown is sparking tensions that never occurred before. Rising property values are for the first time pushing out the residents, often Puerto Ricans. It's a tense time, and a lot of the language used about keeping outsiders away is eerily similar to what whites said when African-Americans moved into their communities. But emotions are too raw to understand the irony.

- One block south of W. Cortland St. you pass under the disused rail tracks that could become the Bloomington Trail, a three-mile urban path that would run from N. Central Park Ave. in the west to the North Branch of the Chicago River in the east, passing through neighborhoods like Humboldt Park and Bucktown. It's a unique opportunity, as the tracks are all elevated on embankments, so you'd be in the city yet above it.

- Cross over to the west side of the street. On the southeast corner of W. Wabansia Ave., Lyman Frank Baum wrote the book that became the movie *The Wizard of Oz* (see Walk 22 for details). Now a small building of public housing, his home looked very much like the nicely restored multi-unit buildings to the south.

- Walk south and cross North Avenue into Humboldt Park. In the late 1800s Chicago had 22 different park commissions, each charged with building and maintaining parks in their section of the city. Exploding populations meant that the commissions on the West Side were at the peak of their powers. The results were three great parks: Garfield, Douglas, and Humboldt. After the commissions were merged in 1934, inertia, ineptitude, and cynicism allowed the parks to fall into a downward spiral. It wasn't until the 1990s that these great civic achievements were given their due—and more importantly, money and care. It's been a long march, but the results in Humboldt Park show that the pay-offs are worth it in a myriad ways. On weekends the park fills with residents enjoying the open space and facilities, the simple aspirations that were the goals when it was built starting in 1871.

Back Story: Chicago's Pearl Necklace

Conceived in the late 1890s, Chicago's boulevards are a 28-mile system of broad, landscaped avenues linking landmark parks. At a time when city streets were pot-holed, narrow, choked with traffic and befouled (see how times change?), the boulevards, stretching in a ring from Diversey Harbor in the north to Jackson Park in the south, were smooth and beautiful. On Sundays, people promenaded in their finest, the cruising of the day. At key points, grand parks like Humboldt served as hubs for the roads. The planners called them a ring of pearls, and soon property developers were adding their own luster. Much of the system suffered in the 20th century, but in recent years the city has done a commendable job of restoring some of the polish. The major parks have been getting long overdue attention, thousands of trees have been planted, and signs erected to mark the system. It's a work in progress, however, and for every success like Logan Blvd., there are still sections like Garfield Blvd. in need of some love.

- Humboldt Blvd. becomes the more serene-sounding Humboldt Dr. in the park. Walk to where it crosses Luis Munõz Marin Dr. Mid-day, there are several lunch trucks here that have some really good food. Look for one with a self-explanatory illustration of a pig on a spit painted on the side. Under the name La Esquina del Sabor, it sells heavenly piles of Puerto Rican pulled pork that translate into one thing: picnic.

- In fact there's even an island named for the activity: Picnic Island. Follow the paths east around the naturalistic East Lagoon and over the bridge to the little island. From here pass through the large and restored 1907 Refectory and Boat House, then curve north over the bridge and east under the road until you're standing near the 1928 Refectory and Field House. It's a chaotic pastiche of European styles that sits overlooking the now-drained West Lagoon (somebody needs to turn on the taps and get the reflective waters back where they should be).

- Walk south along the west side of the newly restored Prairie River, which is one of several features that park superintendent and architect Jens Jensen created in the 1900s as fantasy versions of a naturalized local landscape. On the west are prairie meadows with the requisite profusion of wildflowers blooming in waves through the summer. Midway along the "river," you'll pass a very 21st-century feature: a solar-powered turbine used to pump the water over the features. The path eventually does a little curlicue that neatly encircles Jensen's money-shot, a now-restored small waterfall tumbling over horizontal rocks of limestone in a way Frank Lloyd Wright would have immediately recognized.

- Follow the paths around and back east. South across Division is the half-timbered excess of the 1928 Receptory and Stables, which after many fits and starts is intended to become a Puerto Rican arts center. But set your sights slightly northwest and take time to smell the posies in the concentric rings of the formal rose garden, guarded by two fierce bronze buffalo, which were highlights of the Columbian Exposition.

- Cross N. Humboldt Dr. and follow the park paths to the southeast corner of the park where W. Division St. crosses N. California Ave. Walk east along this vibrant strip of shops and restaurants, which is bracketed by huge stylized Puerto Rican flags arching over the street. Get a taste of local culture at Cafe Colao on the north side past N. Washtenaw Ave. Celebrate finishing your jaunt by choosing from the plethora of tasty flans, famous specialties of the house.

- You can catch a 70 Division bus which will take you east to various El lines.

CONNECTING THE WALKS

The start of this walk links up with the start of Walk 30.

POINTS OF INTEREST

Johnny's Grill 2545 N. Kedzie Ave., 773-278-2215

Lula Cafe 2537 N. Kedzie Blvd., 773-489-9554

El Rinconcito Cubano 3238 W. Fullerton Ave., 773-489-4440

Cafe Colao 2638 W. Division St., 773-276-1780

route summary

1. Start at the Illinois Centennial Monument on Logan Square.
2. Walk south on Kedzie Blvd.
3. At W. Fullerton Ave. turn right and walk west one block.
4. Return to Kedzie Blvd. and continue south.
5. Walk east across Palmer Square.
6. At the east end of Palmer Square, turn right on Humboldt Blvd.
7. Walk south on Humboldt Blvd.
8. Cross North Avenue into Humboldt Park.
9. Follow the paths east around East Lagoon and over the bridge to Picnic Island.
10. Pass through the Refectory and Boat House, then curve north over the bridge and then east under the road to the Refectory and Field House.
11. Walk south along the west side of Prairie River.
12. Follow the paths around the water and back east.
13. Walk northwest to the rose garden.
14. Cross N. Humboldt Dr. and follow the park paths to the southeast corner of the park.

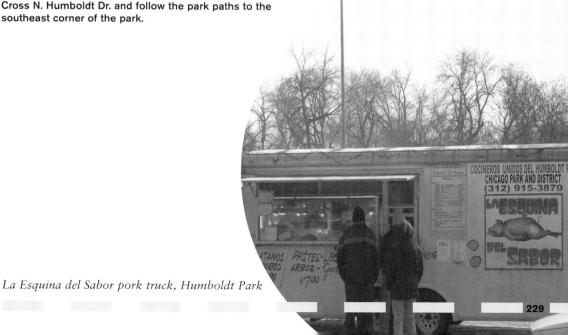

La Esquina del Sabor pork truck, Humboldt Park

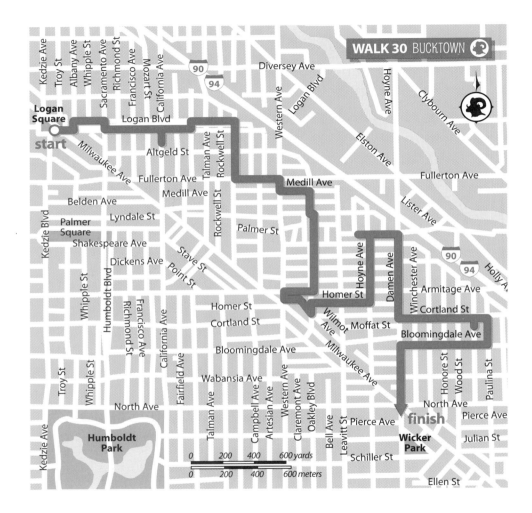

30 BUCKTOWN: GETTING TO KNOW THE GOAT

BOUNDARIES: **Logan Blvd., N. Paulina Ave., W. North Ave., N. Kedzie Ave.**
DISTANCE: **4.9 miles**
PUBLIC TRANSIT: **Blue Line El to Logan Square**

Bucktown may well be Chicago's most-changed community in the last 20 years. In the 1970s it was still a gritty, blue-collar, middle-class enclave; today it's among the most fashionable in town. It's a dynamic mix of new and old that can entertain, repulse, intrigue, and at times even thrill. But despite new homes popping up where sturdy old ones once sat (it seems like just last week), the streets here retain their 100-year-old charm, harkening back to when male goats wandered the streets and the neighborhood gained its name. And amidst a goat-load of glitzy shops and restaurants, there are some very-down-to-earth places. You hardly need walk three blocks before you encounter another classic neighborhood bar. Just northwest of Bucktown, Logan Blvd. runs through one of Chicago's prettiest strips of graystones and other old houses.

- **Start your walk at Logan Square. For this urban expedition, you'll start by going east on one of the richest segments of the Boulevard System.**

- **Wend your way through the traffic nightmare (the designers never could have imagined the SUV-choked streets of today) to the south side of the Logan Square circle and the southwest corner with N. Milwaukee Ave. Look for Wolfbait and B-Girls, a store which lives up to the promise of the name. Representing the best of Bucktown's qualities (hip, funky, smart) as opposed to the worst (pretentious and vacuous), Jenny Stafler and Shirley Novak have created a store with sassy clothes and accessories from local designers.**

- **Cross Milwaukee east. On Sundays there's an indie farmers market on the southeast corner. Not being part of the city system, it has a wider range of goods, including prepared foods, and it takes food stamps.**

- Start on the north side of Logan Blvd. The next three-quarters of a mile is lined with a succession of beautiful graystone houses that present one of the most harmonious man-made vistas in the city. Most date from the early 20th century, a time when Bedford, Indiana limestone had emerged as the material of choice for any Chicago builder that wanted to go one better than brick. Tough yet easily carved, and easily transported by train the 250 miles to the city, its use on Logan Blvd. might as well be a home show for the stuff.

- Past N. Whipple St., 3024 is a multi-unit building that looks like a vast home and is worth the cost of a lease just to sit on the elegant porch. Check out the stained-glass leaded windows at 3016.

- Cross to the south side of Logan Blvd. Between N. Sacramento Ave. and N. Richmond St. is an all-star ensemble cast of graystones (on a street of A-listers). Compare and contrast the details among 2959, 2955, 2951, 2949, and 2947. There's a real big-shouldered brawn to these stolid buildings that can be found for blocks in all directions.

- At N. California Ave., turn south. The first block has several interesting cafes and restaurants, and the exquisite little Provenance Food and Wine store. The carefully selected line-up here offers plenty of picnic potential.

- Return to Logan Blvd. and continue east on the south side. See how many European details you can spot in the melange of limestone over the next two blocks. Start with Romanesque, Gothic, Norman, stopping before you get to Soviet. At the southeast corner of N. Washtenaw Ave. there's a paradigm shift at 2701, which is contemporary with the rest of the street (1907) but has a vaguely Prairie-style motif.

- Cross to the north side and stop at 2656, a once-simple corner brick and wood home that's now a high-end cathedral to kitsch. Everything is lush and plush, from the multi-hued, angel-bedecked bird-bath to the porch griffins to the wiry Eiffel Tower on the side. Christmas decorations here draw crowds.

- Logan Blvd. is cropped by the Kennedy Expressway. Head south on N. Maplewood Ave. and turn east on W. Fullerton Ave. At the intersection with N. Western Ave. (2400 squared in Chicago street-number parlance), Quenchers Saloon has been a mellow venue for great beer since the days when Michelob was considered the good stuff.

- Walk one block south on Western Ave. and then cross into the heart of Bucktown on W. Medill Ave. The neighborhood supposedly takes its name from the male goats that used to wander the streets in the late 1880s when it was an enclave of German and Polish immigrants. The latter also referred to it by the bastardized phrase *Kozie Prery*, which roughly means Goat Prairie, a moniker that actually trumps Bucktown on the fun-o-meter. (And just to stay with the barnyard theme, the area's first name was Holstein.)

- Turn south on N. Oakley Ave. After one block, Senior Citizens Memorial Park puts the cart a bit ahead of the horse in the name department. The street ends at the poll and field house for Holstein Park. Go around the west side and south to the grassy rectangle. There were once three solid sides of sturdy brick two- and three-flats here. Time and gentrification have taken their toll, although the survivors have been restored and still exude a proud sense-of-place (note the arch on 2143 proclaiming its 1890 construction date).

- Continue south on Oakley to W. Armitage Ave. and turn west one block to the rather nasty intersection with N. Western Ave. On the pie-shaped scrap of land at the southwest corner is Margie's, a neighborhood treasure that will help you forget the failure of urban planning outside. Little changed from

3024 Logan Blvd.

the day it opened in 1921, Margie's serves sundaes and other sweet treats; few leave without a 75¢ turtle, just hours old (that would be the candy, by the way, not the critter).

- Make tracks across N. Western Ave. and cut across the parking lot of the McDonald's (averting your eyes from proffers of Happy Meals lest you lose your lunch) to angled N. Wilmot Ave. Go one block southeast to N. Oakley Ave. and turn north for 50 yards to W. Homer St. Now pause, and ask the first person you see if their name is Simpson. That predictable joke out of the way, walk west. On the south side of the street from 2227 to 2247 are nine 1888 princess-sized Queen Anne-style cottages. Although most harmonize, there's a Lucy Ricardo screech at 2247, which hits every false note possible with its insane use of fake rock appliqués. On the other hand, you have to appreciate the individualism, given that so many old gems are disappearing from Bucktown's streets, replaced by new outrages that are the Hummers of the housing world. (Do the owners actually sit around saying: "It was such a charming neighborhood of modest brick homes, that's why we built this steaming pile?")

- Walk to N. Hoyne Ave. and turn north. On the southeast corner with W. Armitage Ave. is the Map Room, another great neighborhood bar. It's got a fine beer selection and décor that's porn for those with wanderlust.

- Continue north for three blocks on Hoyne to yet another ace neighborhood bar. The Charleston is popular with locals who remember when a hummer was somebody who was in a good mood. There's cheap pool and plenty of good chatter.

- Go another two blocks north to W. Webster Ave. The block west has two highlights: at 2121, the 1940s Art Deco façade remains from the funeral parlor that was conveniently located right across from the other highlight: St. Hedwig's Church. Built in 1900 by a Polish congregation, there are still masses said in Polish today. Get too close to the huge bells—say an inch—and you'll be angry.

- Walk east on Webster to N. Damen Ave. and turn south. This is the main commercial drag of Bucktown, and has a huge range of boutiques, cafes, and more. In the first block on the right, number 2148 is notorious as the former office of longtime congressman Dan Rostenkowski, whose career was cut short in 1994 when he was indicted on corruption charges. He ultimately pleaded guilty to lesser charges and spent 15 months in the slammer, joining a long line of Chicago pols who've done time.

● Just across the street is a store dedicated to congress of another kind. G Boutique has all manner of erotic accessories and clothes; you can't miss it as it's pink inside and out.

● Continue south past the many stores (Li'l Guys has great take-away sandwiches, a garden of salads and famous brownies) and cross W. Armitage Ave. At W. Cortland St., turn east and walk four blocks until the hefty backside of St. Mary of the Angels Church comes into view. Circle around to the front facing N. Hermitage Ave. while fully appreciating the dome, which is modeled on no less than St. Peter's Cathedral in Rome. Inside, the fruits of the hard-earned donations of the Polish congregation during the 1910s are lavishly on display.

● One block east on the northeast corner of Cortland and N. Paulina Ave. is an out-crop of cozy establishments, including still another superb neighborhood bar, the Bucktown Pub.

● Walk south one block on N. Paulina St. and then turn west on W. Bloomingdale Ave. Walk five blocks, passing the St. Mary of the Angels bingo hall. At Churchill Park, you may make friends with a schnauzer, as for some dimbulb reason you have to cut through the fenced dog-walking area to get to N. Damen Ave. on the west side. Note the classic modern Bucktown scene as you pass through: starved-to-perfection black-clad owners who are just as boney as their pint-sized pedigreed pooches.

● Assuming you reach Damen with your leg unhumped, turn south, crossing under the disused railroad tracks, which may become the Bloomington Trail (see Walk 29). Walk through another thicket of upscale shops (for the label-obsessed, a stop at Stitch will be like a visit to G Boutique) until you reach the iconic Northwest Tower, on the corner with the same name where Damen meets N. Milwaukee Ave.

● The Blue Line El Damen stop is right here.

CONNECTING THE WALKS

Besides joining Walk 29 at Logan Square, you can join Walk 31 from the end of this walk.

POINTS OF INTEREST

Wolfbait and B-Girls 3131 W. Logan Blvd., 312-698-8685

Provenance Food and Wine 2528 N. California Ave., 773-384-0699

Quenchers Saloon 2401 N. Western Ave., 773-276-9730

Margie's 1960 N. Western Ave., 773-384-1035

Map Room 1949 N. Hoyne Ave., 773-252-7636

Charleston 2076 N. Hoyne Ave., 773-489-4757

G Boutique 2131 N. Damen Ave., 773-235-1234

Li'l Guys 2010 N. Damen Ave., 773-394-6900

Bucktown Pub 1658 W. Cortland Ave., 773-394-9898

Stitch 1723 N. Damen Ave., 773-782-1570

ROUTE SUMMARY

1. Start at Logan Square.
2. Walk east on the north side of Logan Blvd.
3. Cross to the south side of Logan Blvd. at N. Sacramento Ave.
4. At N. California Ave., turn right.
5. Return to Logan Blvd. and continue east on the south side.
6. Cross to the north side..
7. Turn right on N. Maplewood Ave.
8. Turn left on W. Fullerton Ave.
9. Turn right on N. Western Ave. and walk one block.
10. Turn left on W. Medill Ave.

11. Turn right on N. Oakley Ave.

12. Turn right on W. Armitage Ave. and walk to the intersection with N. Western Ave.

13. Cut across the parking lot of the McDonald's to angled N. Wilmot Ave. Turn left.

14. Go one block southeast to N. Oakley Ave. and turn left, walking north for 50 yards to W. Homer St. Turn right.

15. Walk to N. Hoyne Ave. and turn left.

16. Turn right on W. Webster Ave.

17. Turn right on N. Damen Ave.

18. At W. Cortland St., turn left and walk six blocks.

19. Turn right on N. Paulina St.

20. Turn right on W. Bloomingdale Ave. Walk through Churchill Park.

21. Turn left on N. Damen Ave.

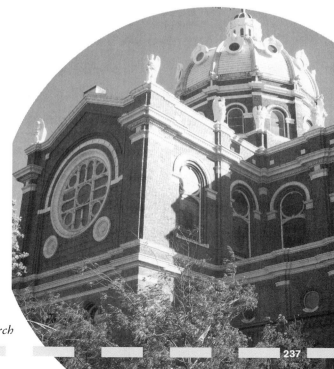

St. Mary of the Angels Church

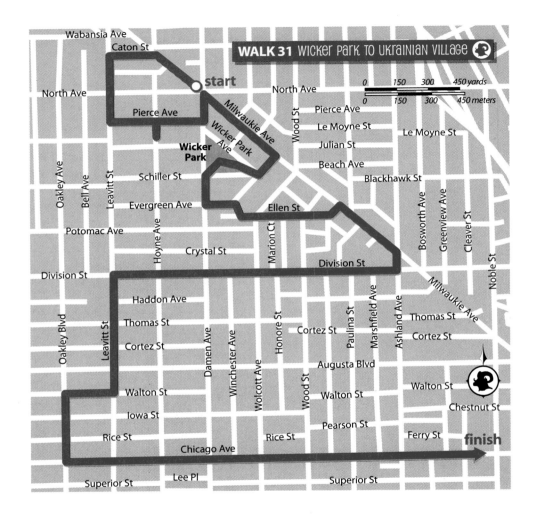

WALK 31 Wicker Park to Ukrainian Village

Wabansia Ave
Caton St
North Ave
Pierce Ave
Milwaukie Ave
Wicker Park Ave
start
North Ave
Pierce Ave
Le Moyne St
Julian St
Beach Ave
Wood St
Le Moyne St
Blackhawk St

0   150   300   450 yards
0   150   300   450 meters

Wicker Park

Oakley Ave
Bell Ave
Leavitt St
Schiller St
Evergreen Ave
Potomac Ave
Hoyne Ave
Crystal St
Marion Ct
Ellen St
Division St
Bosworth Ave
Greenview Ave
Cleaver St

Division St
Haddon Ave
Thomas St
Cortez St
Oakley Blvd
Leavitt St
Damen Ave
Winchester Ave
Wolcott Ave
Honore St
Cortez St
Paulina St
Marshfield Ave
Ashland Ave
Noble St
Milwaukie Ave
Thomas St
Cortez St

Walton St
Iowa St
Rice St
Chicago Ave
Wood St
Augusta Blvd
Walton St
Pearson St
Rice St
Walton St
Chestnut St
Ferry St
finish

Superior St
Lee Pl
Superior St

31 Wicker Park To Ukrainian Village: Walking in Algren's Shoes

BOUNDARIES: W. North Ave., N. Noble St., W. Chicago Ave., N. Western Ave.
DISTANCE: 4½ miles
PUBLIC TRANSIT: Blue Line El to Damen stop

Nelson Algren said loving Chicago is "like loving a woman with a broken nose." Today the once-gritty sidewalks he immortalized in his post-war writings are part of a neighborhood that's had a nose job—and a radical one at that. The twisting streets are still there, but now they're as likely to be lined with Acuras and flowers as with Dodge beaters and snoozing drunks. It's another chapter in the long and varied history of Wicker Park and its smaller sibling Ukrainian Village. A walk here is rich in the legacy of a dozen decades of the city's ups and downs. And even amongst the glitz, Algren would still find plenty that was familiar.

- Start your walk at the Northwest Building at the corner of the same name at the intersection of N. Damen Ave. and N. Milwaukee Ave. This 1929 neighborhood landmark marks the generally agreed-upon W. North Ave. demarcation between Wicker Park and Bucktown. Its 12 stories house many galleries and arts organizations, and it is a hub of the Around the Coyote arts festival every fall.

- Walk northwest two blocks on Milwaukee to W. Caton St. and turn west. This is the heart of what was called the "ethnic Gold Coast" in the late 1800s. Recent immigrants who'd made good built their triumphant homes just blocks away from the modest abodes of their workers. Now of course, with the area being highly desirable, bosses live in the mansions *and* the worker's homes. Highlights on W. Caton include Nos. 2138-2156. This 1891 mini-development features five homes in styles that show much greater variety (2146 is Swiss, 2152 is Renaissance, etc.) than those in your average subdivision, where model differentiation may center on shrub size.

- As you turn south on N. Leavitt St. look amidst the mansions for two upscale vintage apartment buildings at 1644 and 1646 N. Leavitt. You can get a three-bedroom unit here replete with elaborate wood carvings for $1700 per month.

- On the northeast corner with W. Concord Pl., the 1893 house here has been beautifully restored right up to the top of its proud turret.

- Cross W. North Ave. and turn east on W. Pierce Ave. Three carefully restored 1891 houses at 2146, 2150 and 2156 are on the National Register of Historic Places. The owner of a wood-milling company owned the rather unusual house at 2138. Across the street at 2135, detail is piled on detail to where the owners may have needed the serene garden view just to chill out from sensory overload.

- At N. Hoyne St., drop down half a block. At 1520, the 1886 house still has its original figures of carved women. The current owners must be avid horticulturists, judging from the prominent LICK BUSH sign. Across the street, 1521 has wood trim carved to resemble lace.

- Return to Pierce and continue east to N. Damen Ave. and turn north. Cross under the El tracks. On your left is the station, which has been restored to its original (and humble) appearance. On your right, almost under the tracks, is the first of two entrances to the much-vaunted, intimate (473 people max) music venue Double Door.

- Make a sharp turn south on N. Milwaukee Ave. and you'll pass the second entrance to the Double Door—this one for the bands (who in the past have included the Rolling Stones, Poi Dog Pondering, and hundreds more on the way up). Continuing south, Reckless Records and Myopic Books both have names that are slightly pejorative. The former has obscure CDs and plenty of old LPs; the latter has a funky collection full of surprises. Various "second-hand" stores are really ironic boutiques, charging C-notes for junk your parents gleefully unloaded for nickels in 1973.

- At W. Evergreen Ave. turn west. Almost immediately the Mission Christiana Evangelical Church looms into view. Slogans outside may lure you inside if you're ready to question the values that caused you to buy a Land Rover. Directly across the street is the narrow tip of the neighborhood's heart: Wicker Park. The original 1888 fountain has been rebuilt, roses have been planted, the field house spiffed up, and a rather amusing statue of the park's donor, Charles Gustavus Wicker, installed (it's the artistic work of his great-granddaughter). But all is not entirely glittery; there are still a few souls playing cards and feeding squirrels whose luck Nelson Algren could relate to.

- From the west side of Wicker Park, walk south on N. Damen Ave. for a short block and turn east on W. Evergreen Ave. Nelson Algren lived for almost 20 years in the rather elegant brick three-flat at 1958. Wicker Park's Division St. and Milwaukee Ave. were at the heart of his gritty urban realm, which inspired masterpieces such as *The Neon Wilderness*. He once said: "People ask me why I don't write about nature or the suburbs. If a writer could write the truth about one Chicago street, that would be a good life's work."

- From Algren's apartment, walk east 50 yards until you see an alley heading south. Walk into the alley and compare the two homes that straddle it: 1945 and 1947. The former is original right down to its carefully detailed brick ornamentation. The latter is new, with clichéd limestone-esque mullions and garish white grout that screams "this little piggy built his house out of brick!"

- The alley ends after 50 yards. Take a gentle left east, skipping the alley on the immediate left and opting for the stub-end of W. Ellen St. Walk east for about 400 yards on Ellen until you reach the El tracks, then follow the short spur under the tracks to N. Milwaukee Ave. In comparison to the hipster chunk of Milwaukee up by North Ave., this stretch is much more proletarian in its tastes. Here the second-hand stores are really second-hand stores; the cheap junk is cheap. The well-off people who now live in Wicker Park drive elsewhere to shop, while the poor people they displaced return to the old 'hood. Should life's aggravations—such as the humor in this book—have you pulling your hair out, the Heads and Threads Boutique will sell you a wig in any color you wish.

- At the resolutely ungentrified landmark intersection of N. Milwaukee Ave., N. Ashland Ave. and W. Division St., curl around and head west on Division. The one-mile strip from here almost to W. Western Ave. has changed to such an extent in the last 10 years that Algren would be hard-pressed to recognize it. Old apartments have been converted to condos, some new condos have been built to look like old apartments, and other new condos have been built to look like nothing in the city. You can get a two-bedroom unit for $600,000 (including granite countertops).

- In the 1940s, Division St. was known as the Polish Broadway for its ethnic mix (or lack of it). Algren set *The Man With the Golden Arm* here, Frankie Machine and his wife Sophie battling their addictions amidst Division Street's temptations. The novel won the National Book Award in 1950, and Otto Preminger made it into a movie starring an unusually restrained Frank Sinatra. Although there's no sign saying Algren slept here, the gritty Gold Star Bar near the southeast corner of N. Wood St. dates from his era, and is four blocks from his flat.

- And all is not tofu and Stella beer. On the northwest corner of N. Wood St., Phyllis' Musical Inn predates all the recent upheavals. For a couple of bucks you can hear top garage bands ripping into their own songs. On Sundays and Mondays, things slow way down for jazz. Across Division St. is another institution that Algren would probably have approved of: Splat Flats. To the casual observer it looks like L Miller and Son Lumber Co., but in the spaces above and behind the wood are 28 studios for artists ranging from painters to the highest practitioners of the arts, writers. Rents average $200 a month; these spaces are much sought after by Chicago's large but often hidden artistic community.

- Division Street's sidewalks are extra wide; the reasons why are lost, but they do a good job of accommodating outdoor cafes—none trendier than Crust. Near N. Hoyne Ave., it's for those who wanted a Melrose Ave. joint in L.A. but forgot to fly over and ended up in Chicago instead. Nearby you can get a scooter, and if we'd looked hard enough, probably somewhere to get a tiny, trendy dog as well.

- At N. Leavitt St., turn south—and not a moment too soon. Just west is the horrific 1975 hulk of St. Mary of Nazareth Hospital. About the only thing that can be said about it is that at least once the sick are inside, their recovery can't be impeded by seeing it from the outside.

- After a short block, the weathered white of Holy Trinity Russian Orthodox Church sits quietly on the corner. It was an 1899 commission for Louis Sullivan, who infused traditional designs with his own esthetic. From some angles it actually looks like a sitting, yet alert dog—but nowhere near as ugly as the tiny ones at the cafes back around the corner.

- Walk south on Leavitt, crossing west to N. Oakley Blvd. on W. Walton St. These tidy blocks are the heart of Ukrainian Village, an ethnic enclave that had as many as

30,000 Ukrainians living there in 1930, but only 2,000 by the year 2000. Just past W. Iowa St., St. Nickolas Ukrainian Catholic Church dates from 1915, and has especially rich mosaics above the doors. Note the Madonna and child.

- At W. Chicago Ave., a few Ukrainian businesses hang on. Look for posters in the windows touting visiting Ukrainian rock bands. Look south down S. Oakley to see the 1975 Sts. Volodymyr and Olha Church, one of the magnets that keeps drawing back the Chicagoland Ukrainian diaspora.

- Walk east on W. Chicago Ave. At the southeast corner of N. Leavitt St. is a metaphor for the entire neighborhood. Tuman's is a beautifully restored 1890's pub with a family-friendly menu. In the early 1990's it was known by its full name: Tuman's Alcohol Abuse Center. The original interior was hidden under a layer of filth, the beer (in cans) was cheap, and one night when I was there, I spotted a line of roaches marching up my friend's barstool. Who knew she could move so quick? Note the minuscule A. A. C. on the sign today, a vague nod to the past.

- For a taste of the neighborhood's roots, pick up some Polish pierogi at Kasia's. The biggest skeptic will be converted by these tasty filled pockets.

- East of N. Damen Ave., the street becomes a mix of new places redolent with gentrification, and older Hispanic merchants. Two long-running Mexican restaurants each have their strengths: Tecalitlan has sublime beans and tangy al pastor burritos, while Taco Veloz has a kitchen right up front, good pickled vegetables, and torts oozing with creamy avocado. Just east, the horse mounted over the sidewalk signals you've found Acala's Western Wear, a store that brings a Tex-Mex flavor to all things cowpoke. Start with the 10,000 pairs of boots and move right on through to the bolo ties.

- Past N. Ashland Ave., look for Mercury Cafe on the south side of the street, just before N. Armour St. It's a vast former discount store, and little has changed, although the girdle counter is gone for good. The vibe here defines funky, the coffee is organic, and the politics left-of-center. There's free wi-fi and quite a few freelancers working away at the tables, getting a respite from shooing the cat off the keyboard at home.

- Finish your walk in a melting pot of Chicago nightlife. One short block north of W. Chicago Ave. on the northeast corner with W. Fry St., the Chipp Inn is a modern version of the Chicago corner bar: unpretentious and friendly, where you can argue the merits of the Cubs and your alderman. Follow Fry west and around back to Chicago Ave.; Five Star on the northeast corner is a popular bar and grill with good burgers, booths and tables outside. Finally, just east on the other side of N. Bishop St. is Sonotheque, a Euro-style club without the Euro-trash. It's glam without a surfeit of posers, and the deejays are spot on.

- End your walk by hopping aboard the 66 Chicago bus to El lines east, and consider this bit of advice from Nelson Algren: "Never play cards with a man called Doc. Never eat at a place called Mom's. Never sleep with a woman whose troubles are worse than your own."

POINTS OF INTEREST

Double Door 1572 N. Milwaukee Ave., 773-489-3160

Reckless Records 1532 N. Milwaukee Ave., 773-235-3727

Myopic Books 1468 N. Milwaukee Ave., 773-862-4882

Heads and Threads Boutique 1254 N. Milwaukee Ave., 773-235-1190

Phyllis' Musical Inn 1800 W. Division St., 773-486-9862

Gold Star Bar 1755 W. Division St., 773-227-8700

Crust 2056 W. Division St., 773-235-5511

Kasia's 2101 W. Chicago Ave., 773-486-6163

Tecalitlan 1814 W. Chicago Ave., 773-384-4285

Taco Veloz 1745 W. Chicago Ave., 312-738-0363

Acala's 1733 W. Chicago Ave., 312-226-0152

Mercury Cafe 1505 W. Chicago Ave., 312-455-9924

Chipp Inn 832 N. Greenview Ave., 312-421-9052

Five Star 1424 W. Chicago Ave., 312-850-2555

Sonotheque 1444 W. Chicago Ave., 312-226-7600

route summary

1. Start at the Northwest Building at the intersection of N. Damen Ave. and N. Milwaukee Ave.
2. Walk northwest two blocks on Milwaukee.
3. Turn left on W. Caton St.
4. Turn left on N. Leavitt St.
5. Turn left on W. Pierce Ave.
6. At N. Hoyne St., drop down half a block.
7. Return to Pierce and continue east.
8. Turn left on N. Damen Ave.
9. Make a sharp turn south on N. Milwaukee Ave.
10. At W. Evergreen Ave. turn right.
11. From the west side of Wicker Park, turn left and walk south on N. Damen Ave.
12. Turn left on W. Evergreen Ave.
13. Go through an alley heading south for 50 yards.
14. Take a gentle left east, skipping the alley on the immediate left and opting for the stub-end of W. Ellen St.
15. Walk east for about 400 yards on Ellen until you reach the El tracks, then follow the short spur under the tracks to N. Milwaukee Ave.
16. Turn right on Milwaukee.
17. At the intersection of N. Milwaukee Ave., N. Ashland Ave. and W. Division St., curl around and head west on Division.
18. At N. Leavitt St., turn left.
19. Turn right on W. Walton St.
20. Turn left on N. Oakley Blvd.
21. At W. Chicago Ave. turn left.

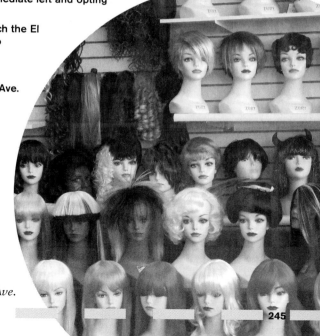

Wigged out on Milwaukee Ave.

Appendix 1: WALKS BY THEME

The walks listed below have at least one major component that fits the theme.

ARCHITECTURE

Hyde Park (Walk 3)
Kenwood (Walk 4)
Pullman (Walk 7)
Oak Park (Walk 9)
South Loop and Near South Side (Walk 13)
Millennium Park to Navy Pier (Walk 16)
The Loop and Printer's Row (Walk 17)
The Chicago River (Walk 19)
Magnificent Mile and Streeterville (Walk 20)
Gold Coast and Old Town (Walk 21)
South Michigan Ave. (Walk 23)

CLASSIC CHICAGO NEIGHBORHOODS

Just the name evokes a picture, a mood, a sense of place.

South Shore (Walk 1)
Kenwood (Walk 4)
Pullman (Walk 7)
Beverly and Morgan Park (Walk 8)
Bronzeville and Bridgeport (Walk 10)
Little Italy (Walk 12)
Pilsen (Walk 14)
Chinatown (Walk 15)
Gold Coast and Old Town (Walk 21)
Lincoln Park (Walk 22)
Lake View to Wrigleyville (Walk 24)
Uptown and Andersonville (Walk 25)
North Branch and Lincoln Square (Walk 27)

Devon Avenue and North Park (Walk 28)
Logan Square and Humboldt Park (Walk 29)
Bucktown (Walk 30)
Wicker Park and Ukrainian Village (Walk 31)

DINING AND ENTERTAINMENT

West Loop (Walk 11)
Little Italy (Walk 12)
River North (Walk 18)
Magnificent Mile and Streeterville (Walk 20)
Gold Coast and Old Town (Walk 21)
Lincoln Park (Walk 22)
Lake View to Wrigleyville (Walk 24)
Uptown and Andersonville (Walk 25)
North Branch and Lincoln Square (Walk 27)
Devon Avenue and North Park (Walk 28)
Bucktown (Walk 30)
Wicker Park and Ukrainian Village (Walk 31)

LAKEFRONT

South Shore (Walk 1)
Burnham Park (Walk 5)
Grant Park to Northerly Island (Walk 6)
Millennium Park to Navy Pier (Walk 16)
Magnificent Mile and Streeterville (Walk 20)
Lincoln Park (Walk 22)
Uptown and Andersonville (Walk 25)
Belmont to Montrose (Walk 26)

HISTOrY

Every walk in this book has history in it; these have significant history.

Washington Park and Jackson Park (Walk 2)
Hyde Park (Walk 3)
Bronzeville and Bridgeport (Walk 10)
South Loop and Near South Side (Walk 13)
The Loop and Printer's Row (Walk 17)
River North (Walk 18)
South Michigan Ave. (Walk 23)

SHOPPING

You can always buy something (sometimes from a guy in an alley); these walks pass a lot of noteworthy shops.

River North (Walk 18)
Magnificent Mile and Streeterville (Walk 20)
Gold Coast and Old Town (Walk 21)
Lincoln Park (Walk 22)

GreaT ParKs

Washington Park and Jackson Park (Walk 2)
Burnham Park (Walk 5)
Grant Park to Northerly Island (Walk 6)
Millennium Park to Navy Pier (Walk 16)
Lincoln Park (Walk 22)
Logan Square and Humboldt Park (Walk 29)

UrBaN BeauTY

Not a park, not the lakefront, but damn nice anyway.

Hyde Park (Walk 3)
Kenwood (Walk 4)
Beverly and Morgan Park (Walk 8)
Oak Park (Walk 9)
The Loop and Printer's Row (Walk 17)
The Chicago River (Walk 19)
Magnificent Mile and Streeterville (Walk 20)
Gold Coast and Old Town (Walk 21)
South Michigan Ave. (Walk 23)
Belmont to Montrose (Walk 26)
Devon Avenue and North Park (Walk 28)
Bucktown (Walk 30)

UrBaN GriT

Where you can still get a whiff of the "city of big shoulders."

Pullman (Walk 7)
Bronzeville and Bridgeport (Walk 10)
West Loop (Walk 11)
Little Italy (Walk 12)
South Loop and Near South Side (Walk 13)
Pilsen (Walk 14)
Logan Square and Humboldt Park (Walk 29)
Wicker Park and Ukrainian Village (Walk 31)

Appendix 2: POINTS OF INTEREST

architecture and historical landmarks

Auditorium Theater www.auditoriumtheater.org, 50 E. Congress Pkwy., 312-922-2110 (Walk 23)

Barack Obama house Hyde Park Blvd and S. Greenwood Ave. (Walk 4)

Bubbly Creek (Walk 10)

Burnham Park (Walk 5)

Carbon and Carbide Building 30 N. Michigan Ave. (Walk 23)

Carl Sandburg house 4646 N. Hermitage Ave. (Walk 27)

Charnley House 1365 N. Astor St., 312-915-0105 (Walk 21)

Chicago Board of Trade Building 141 W. Jackson Blvd. (Walk 17)

Chicago Hilton and Towers www.chicagohilton.com, 720 S. Michigan Ave., 312-922-4400 (Walk 23)

Crilly Court (Walk 21)

Ernest Hemingway Birthplace and Museum www.ehfop.org, 339 Oak Park Ave. and 200 Oak Park Ave., 708-524-5383 (Walk 9)

Fisher Building 343 S. Dearborn St. (Walk 17)

Frank Lloyd Wright Home and Studio www.wrightplus.org, 951 Chicago Ave., 708-848-1976 (Walk 9)

Graceland Cemetery 4001 N. Clark St., 773-525-1105 (Walk 26)

Grant Park (Walk 6 and Walk 23)

Haymarket statue W. Randolph St. and N. Des Plaines Ave. (Walk 11)

Hotel Florence/Pullman State Historic Site www.pullman-museum.org, 1111 S. Florence Ave., 773-660-2342 (Walk 7)

Humboldt Park (Walk 29)

Hyatt Center 71 S. Wacker Dr. (Walk 17)

Illinois Institute of Technology www.iit.edu, 3300 S. Federal St., 312-567-3000 (Walk 10)

Jane Addams Hull House Museum 800 S. Halsted St., 312-413-5353 (Walk 12)

John Hancock Center 875 N. Michigan Ave. (Walk 20)

John J. Glessner House www.glessnerhouse.org, 1800 S. Prairie Ave., 312-326-1480 (Walk 13)

Logan Square 2600 N. Milwaukee Ave. (Walk 29 and Walk 30)

Marina City 300 N. State St. (Walk 19)

Merchandise Mart 320 N. Wells St. (Walk 19)

Michigan Ave. Bridge (Walk 20)

Millennium Park (Walk 16)

Monadnock Building 53 W. Jackson Blvd. (Walk 17)

Museum of Science and Industry www.msichicago.org, W. 57th St. and Lake Shore Dr., 773-684-1414 (Walk 2)

Nelson Algren flat 1958 W. Evergreen Ave. (Walk 31)

Picasso sculpture Daley Plaza (Walk 17)

Reliance Building (a.k.a. Hotel Burnham, www.burnhamhotel.com, 312-782-1111) 1 W. Washington St. (Walk 17)

Robie House www.wrightplus.org, 5757 S. Woodlawn Ave., 708-848-1976 (Walk 3)

Sears Tower 233 S. Wacker Dr. (Walk 17)

Stephen A. Douglas Tomb and Memorial (Walk 5)

Tribune Tower 435 N. Michigan Ave. (Walk 20)

Trump International Hotel and Tower www.trumpchicago.com, 401 N. Wabash St. (Walk 19)

Union Station 210 South Canal St. (Walk 19)

Uptown Theater 4816 N. Broadway (Walk 25)

W. Kinzie St. Bridge (Walk 19)

Willie Dixon's Blues Heaven Foundation 2120 S. Michigan Ave., 312-808-1286 (Walk 13)

Wrigley Building 400 N. Michigan Ave. (Walk 19)

CHUrCHes

Holy Family Church 1080 W. Roosevelt Rd. (Walk 12)

Holy Name Cathedral 735 N. State St. (Walk 18)

Holy Trinity Russian Orthodox Church 1121 N. Leavitt St. (Walk 31)

St. Adalbert Church 1650 W. 17th St. (Walk 14)

St. Mary of the Angels Church 1850 N. Hermitage Ave. (Walk 30)

St. Paul's Church 2127 W. 22nd Pl. (Walk 14)

St. Procopius Church 1641 S. Allport St. (Walk 14)

St. Therese Catholic Church 218 W. Alexander St. (Walk 15)

Unity Temple 875 Lake St., 708-383-8873 (Walk 9)

CULTUraL anD eDUCaTIONaL INSTITUTIONS

Auditorium Theater www.auditoriumtheater.org, 50 E. Congress Pkwy., 312-922-2110 (Walk 23)

Beverly Arts Center www.beverlyartcenter.org, 2407 W. 111th St., 773-445-3838 (Walk 8)

Center on Halsted 3656 N. Halsted St., 773-472-6469 (Walk 24)

Chicago Architecture Foundation www.architecture.org, 224 S. Michigan Ave., 312-922-3432 (Walk 23)

Chicago Cultural Center 78 E. Washington St., 312-744-6630 (Walk 23)

Chicago Shakespeare Theater www.chicagoshakes.com, 312-595-5600 (Walk 16)

Chicago Symphony Orchestra www.cso.org, 220 S. Michigan Ave., 312-294-3000 (Walk 23)

City of Chicago Tourism Office Water Tower Pumping Station, 163 E. Pearson Ave., 877-244-2246 (Walk 20)

Columbia College www.colum.edu, 600 S. Michigan Ave., 312-663-1600 (Walk 23)

Ernest Hemingway Birthplace and Museum www.ehfop.org, 339 Oak Park Ave. and 200 Oak Park Ave., 708-524-5383 (Walk 9)

Frank Lloyd Wright Home and Studio www.wrightplus.org, 951 Chicago Ave., 708-848-1976 (Walk 9)

Gene Siskel Film Center 164 N. State St., 312-846-2800 (Walk 17)

Historic Pullman Visitor Center www.pullmanil.org, 11141 S. Cottage Grove Ave., 773-785-8901 (Walk 7)

Hubbard St. Dance Centre www.hubbardstreetdance.org, 1147 W. Jackson Blvd., 312-850-9744 (Walk 11)

Illinois Institute of Technology www.iit.edu, 3300 S. Federal St., 312-567-3000 (Walk 10)

John Hancock Center Observatory 875 N. Michigan Ave., 312-751-3681 (Walk 20)

John J. Glessner House www.glessnerhouse.org, 1800 S. Prairie Ave., 312-326-1480 (Walk 13)

Lincoln Park Zoo www.lpzoo.com, 2001 N. Clark St., 312-742-2000 (Walk 22)

Navy Pier www.navypier.com, 312-595-7437 (Walk 16)

Newberry Library 60 W. Walton St., 312-255-3504 (Walk 18)

North Park Village Nature Center 5801 N. Pulaski Rd., 312-744-5472 (Walk 28)

Oak Park Library 834 Lake St., 708-383-8200 (Walk 9)

Oak Park Visitors Center 158 Forest Ave., 708-848-1500 (Walk 9)

Old Town School of Folk Music www.oldtownschool.org, 4544 N. Lincoln Ave., 773-751-3398 (Walk 27)

Roosevelt University www.roosevelt.edu, 430 S. Michigan Ave., 312-341-3500 (Walk 23)

Sears Tower Skydeck 233 S. Wacker Dr., 312-875-9447 (Walk 17)

South Shore Cultural Center 7059 S. South Shore Dr., 773-256-0149 (Walk 1)

University of Chicago www.uchicago.edu, 801 S. Ellis Ave., 773-702-1234 (Walk 3)

University of Illinois at Chicago www.uic.edu, 1200 West Harrison St., 312-996-7000 (Walk 12)

Victory Gardens Theater Greenhouse 2257 N. Lincoln Ave., 773-871-3000 (Walk 22)

eaTING aND DrINKING

17/West at the Berghoff 17 W. Adams St., 312-427-3170 (Walk 17)

Al's No. 1 Italian Beef 1079 W. Taylor St., 312-226-4017 (Walk 12)

Andie's 5253 N. Clark St., 773-784-8616 (Walk 25)

Annette's Homemade Italian Ice 2009 N. Bissell St., 773-868-9000 (Walk 22)

Artopolis Bakery Cafe Agora 306 S. Halsted St., 312-559-9000 (Walk 11)

Arya Bhavan 2508 W. Devon Ave., 773-274-5800 (Walk 28)

Berlin 954 W. Belmont Ave., 773-348-4975 (Walk 24)

Big Chicks 5024 N. Sheridan Rd., 773-728-5511 (Walk 25)

Bijan's Bistro 633 N. State St., 312-202-1904 (Walk 18)

Billy Goat Tavern 430 N. Michigan Ave. (lower level), 312-222-1525 (Walk 20)

Brasserie Ruhlmann 500 W. Superior St., 312-494-1900 (Walk 18)

Brehon Pub 731 N. Wells St., 312-642-1071 (Walk 18)

Bridgeport Coffee Company 3101 S. Morgan St., 773-247-9950 (Walk 10)

Bruna's Ristorante 2424 S. Oakley Ave., 773-254-5550 (Walk 14)

Bucktown Pub 1658 W. Cortland Ave., 773-394-9898 (Walk 30)

Café Luna 1742 W. 99th St, 773-239-8990 (Walk 8)

Cafe Mestizo 1646 W. 18th St., 312-421-5920 (Walk 14)

Café Society 1801 S. Indiana Ave., 312-842-4210 (Walk 13)

Cal Harbor Restaurant 546 E. 115th St, 773-264-5436 (Walk 7)

Casey's Corner 2733 W. Devon Ave. (Walk 28)

Chalkboard 4343 N. Lincoln Ave., 773-477-7144 (Walk 27)

Charleston 2076 N. Hoyne Ave., 773-489-4757 (Walk 30)

Charlie Trotter's 816 W. Armitage Ave., 773-248-6228 (Walk 22)

Chicago Brauhaus 4732 N. Lincoln Ave., 773-784-4444 (Walk 27)

Chicago Diner 3411 N. Halsted St., 773-935-6696 (Walk 24)

Chipp Inn 832 N. Greenview Ave., 312-421-9052 (Walk 31)

Chiu Quon Bakery and Cafe 2242 S. Wentworth Ave., 312-225-6608 (Walk 15)

Clark St. Ale House 742 N. Clark St., 312-642-9253 (Walk 18)

Coq d'Or Drake Hotel 140 E. Walton Pl., 312-787-1431 (Walk 20)

Crust 2056 W. Division St., 773-235-5511 (Walk 31)

Demera Ethiopian 4801 N. Broadway, 773-334-8787 (Walk 25)

Dollop Coffee Co. 4181 N. Clarendon St., 773-755-1955 (Walk 26)

Donald's Hot Dogs 2325 S. Western Ave., 773-254-7777 (Walk 14)

Dubliner 10910 S. Western Ave, 773-238-0784 (Walk 8)

Dunkin' Donuts 3200 N. Clark St., 773-477-3636 (Walk 24)

El Rinconcito Cubano 3238 W. Fullerton Ave., 773-489-4440 (Walk 29)

Emperor's Choice 2238 S. Wentworth Ave., 312-225-8800 (Walk 15)

Exchange Cafe 7201 S. Exchange Ave., 773-336-8592 (Walk 1)

Five Star 1424 W. Chicago Ave., 312-850-2555 (Walk 31)

Fontano's Subs 20 E. Jackson Blvd., 312-663-3061 (Walk 17)

Frontera Fresco Macy's 111 N. State St., 312-781-4483 (Walk 17)

Funky Buddha 728 W. Grand Ave., 312-666-1695 (Walk 11)

Garrett Popcorn 2 W. Jackson Blvd., 312-360-1108 (Walk 17)

Gibson's 1028 N. Rush St., 312-266-8999 (Walk 21)

Gingerman 3740 N. Clark St., 773-549-2050 (Walk 24)

Gold Star Bar 1755 W. Division St., 773-227-8700 (Walk 31)

Good Morgan 2948 W. Devon Ave., 773-764-8115 (Walk 28)

Guthrie's 1300 W. Addison Ave., 773-477-2900 (Walk 24)

Hidden Pearl Art Cafe 1060 E. 47th St., 773-285-1211 (Walk 4)

Hopleaf 5148 N. Clark St., 773-334-9851 (Walk 25)

Huettenbar 4721 N. Lincoln Ave., 773-561-2507 (Walk 27)

ImprovOlympics 3541 N. Clark St., 773-880-0199 (Walk 24)

Japonais 600 W. Chicago Ave., 312-822-9600 (Walk 18)

Jilly's 1007 N. Rush St., 312-664-1001 (Walk 21)

Jimmy Jamm Sweet Potato Pies 1742 W. 99th St., 773-239-8990 (Walk 8)

Jim's 1250 S. Union Ave., 312-733-7820 (Walk 12)

Johnny's Grill 2545 N. Kedzie Ave., 773-278-2215 (Walk 29)

Jury's Food and Drink 4337 N. Lincoln Ave., 773-935-2255 (Walk 27)

Kamdar Plaza 2646 W. Devon Ave., 773-338-8100 (Walk 28)

Kasey's Tavern 701 S. Dearborn St., 312-427-7992 (Walk 17)

Kasia's 2101 W. Chicago Ave., 773-486-6163 (Walk 31)

Kit Kat Lounge 3700 N. Halsted St., 773-525-1111 (Walk 24)

Kristoffer's Cafe and Bakery 1733 S. Halsted St., 312-829-4150 (Walk 14)

La Fontanella 2414 S. Oakley Ave., 773-927-5249 (Walk 14)

Li'l Guys 2010 N. Damen Ave., 773-394-6900 (Walk 30)

Lula Cafe 2537 N. Kedzie Blvd., 773-489-9554 (Walk 29)

Lutz Cafe and Pastry Shop 2458 W. Montrose Ave., 773-478-7785 (Walk 27)

Manny's 1141 S. Jefferson St., 312-939-2855 (Walk 12)

Map Room 1949 N. Hoyne Ave., 773-252-7636 (Walk 30)

Margie's 1960 N. Western Ave., 773-384-1035 (Walk 30)

Mario's Italian Lemonade 1068 W. Taylor St. (Walk 12)

Market St. Inn 955 W. Randolph St., 312-829-9170 (Walk 11)

McNally's 11136 S. Western Ave., 773-779-6202 (Walk 8)

Melrose Restaurant 3233 N. Broadway, 773-327-2060 (Walk 26)

Mercury Cafe 1505 W. Chicago Ave., 312-455-9924 (Walk 31)

Miceli's Deli 2448 S. Oakley Ave., 773-847-6873 (Walk 14)

Mitchell's 3356 S. Halsted St., 773-927-6073 (Walk 10)

Mughal Bakery 6348 N. Maplewood Ave., 773-761-9660 (Walk 28)

Murphy's Bleachers 3655 N. Sheffield Ave., 773-281-5356 (Walk 24)

Nookies Tree 3344 N. Halsted St., 773-248-9888 (Walk 24)

North Pond 2610 N. Cannon Dr., 773-477-5845 (Walk 22)

Old Town Ale House 219 W. North Ave., 312-944-7020 (Walk 21)

Opera 1301 S. Wabash Ave., 312-461-0161 (Walk 13)

Pan Hellenic Pastry Shop 324 S. Halsted St., 312-454-1886 (Walk 11)

Parthenon 314 S. Halsted St., 312-726-2407 (Walk 11)

Pasta Shoppe and Cafe 116 N. Oak Park Ave., 708-763-0600 (Walk 9)

Pie Hole Pizza 739 N. Halsted St., 773-525-8888 (Walk 24)

Pizzeria Uno 29 E. Ohio St., 312-321-1000 (Walk 18)

Provenance Food and Wine 2528 N. California Ave., 773-384-0699 (Walk 30)

Pullman's Pub 611 E. 113th St., 773-568-0264 (Walk 7)

Quenchers Saloon 2401 N. Western Ave., 773-276-9730 (Walk 30)

Ramova's Grill 3510 S. Halsted St., 773-847-9058 (Walk 10)

Restaurante Nuevo Leon 1515 W. 18th St., 312-421-1517 (Walk 14)

Roscoe's 3356 N. Halsted St., 773-281-3355 (Walk 24)

Rosebud 1550 W. Taylor St., 312-755-1777 (Walk 12)

Scafuri Bakery 1337 W. Taylor St., 312-733-8881 (Walk 12)

Sterch's 2238 N. Lincoln Ave., 773-281-2653 (Walk 22)

Sukhadia's 2559 W. Devon Ave., 773-338-5400 (Walk 28)

Taco Veloz 1745 W. Chicago Ave., 312-738-0363 (Walk 31)

Tastee Freez 2815 W. Armitage Ave., 773-252-1464 (Walk 29)

Tecalitlan 1814 W. Chicago Ave., 773-384-4285 (Walk 31)

The Closet 3333 N. Broadway, 773-477-8533 (Walk 26)

The Pump Room 1301 N. State Pkwy., 312-266-0360 (Walk 21)

Three Happiness 209 W. Cermak Rd., 312-842-1964 (Walk 15)

Tufano's Vernon Park Tap 1073 W. Vernon Park Pl., 312-733-3393 (Walk 12)

Twin Anchors 1655 N. Sedgwick St., 312-266-1616 (Walk 21)

Whirlaway Lounge 3224 W. Fullerton Ave., 773-276-6809 (Walk 29)

Wild Hare 3530 N. Clark St., 773-327-4273 (Walk 24)

Wishbone 1001 W. Washington Blvd., 312-850-2663 (Walk 11)

Won Kow 2237 S. Wentworth Ave., 312-842-7500 (Walk 15)

entertainment and nightlife

Annoyance Theater 4830 N. Broadway, 773-561-4665 (Walk 25)

Aragon Ballroom 1106 W. Lawrence Ave., 773-989-0675 (Walk 25)

New Checkerboard Lounge 5201 S. Harper Ct., 773-684-1472 (Walk 4)

Chicago White Sox chicago.whitesox.mlb.com, 333 W. 35th St., 312-674-1000 (Walk 10)

ComedySportz 929 W. Belmont Ave., 312-733-6000 (Walk 24)

Double Door 1572 N. Milwaukee Ave., 773-489-3160 (Walk 31)

Green Mill 4802 N. Broadway, 773-878-5552 (Walk 25)

Music Box 3733 N. Southport Ave., 773-871-6604 (Walk 24)

Phyllis' Musical Inn 1800 W. Division St., 773-486-9862 (Walk 31)

Riviera Theater 4746 N. Broadway, 773-275-6800 (Walk 25)

Sonotheque 1444 Chicago Ave., 312-226-7600 (Walk 31)

Sydney R. Marovitz Golf Course Lincoln Park 3600 N. Recreation Dr., 312-245-0909 (Walk 26)

The Pub Ida Noyes Hall 1212 E. 59th St., 773-702-9737 (Walk 3)

Woodlawn Tap 1172 E. 55th St., 773-643-5516 (Walk 3)

Wrigley Field 1060 W. Addison St. (Walk 24)

galleries and museums

Adler Planetarium www.adlerplanetarium.org, 1300 S. Lake Shore Dr., 312-922-7827 (Walk 6)

Art Institute of Chicago www.artic.edu, 111 S. Michigan Ave., 312-443-3600 (Walk 23)

Bridgehouse and Chicago River Museum 376 N. Michigan Ave., 312-977-0227 (Walk 19)

Chicago Children's Museum 700 E. Grand Avenue, #127, 312-527-1000 (Walk 16)

Chicago Cultural Center 78 E. Washington St., 312-744-6630 (Walk 23)

Chicago History Museum 1601 N. Clark St., 312-642-4600 (Walk 21)

Chinese-American Museum of Chicago 238 W. 23rd St., 312-949-1000 (Walk 15)

DuSable Museum of African American History www.dusablemuseum.org, 740 E. 56th Pl., 773-947-0600 (Walk 2)

EXP Gallery 726 W. 18th St., 847-217-7520 (Walk 14)

Field Museum www.fieldmuseum.org, 1400 S. Lake Shore Dr., 312-922-9410 (Walk 6)

Hidden Pearl Art Cafe 1060 E. 47th St., 773-285-1211 (Walk 4)

Jane Addams Hull House Museum 800 S. Halsted St., 312-413-5353 (Walk 12)

Judy Saslow Gallery 300 W. Superior St., 312-943-0530 (Walk 18)

McCormick Tribune Freedom Museum 445 N. Michigan Ave., 312-222-4860 (Walk 20)

Museum of Contemporary Art 220 E. Chicago Ave., 312-280-2660 (Walk 20)

Museum of Contemporary Photography www.mocp.org, 600 S. Michigan Ave., 312-663-5554 (Walk 23)

Museum of Science and Industry www.msichicago.org, W. 57th St. and Lake Shore Dr., 773-684-1414 (Walk 2)

National Italian American Sports Hall of Fame 1431 W. Taylor St., 312-226-5566 (Walk 12)

National Vietnam Veterans Art Museum www.nvvam.org, 1801 S. Indiana Ave., 312-326-0270 (Walk 13)

Notebaert Nature Museum www.chias.org, 2430 N. Cannon Dr., 773-755-5100 (Walk 22)

Oriental Institute 1155 E. 58th St., 773-702-9514 (Walk 3)

Ridge Historical Society www.ridgehistoricalsociety.org, 10621 S. Seeley Ave., 773-881-1675 (Walk 8)

Shedd Aquarium www.sheddaquarium.org, 1200 S. Lake Shore Dr., 312-939-2426 (Walk 6)

Spertus Institute of Jewish Studies 610 S. Michigan Ave., 312-322-1700 (Walk 23)

Stephen Daiter Gallery 311 W. Superior St., 312-787-3350 (Walk 18)

HOTELS

Ambassador East Hotel www.theambassadoreasthotel.com, 1301 N. State Pkwy., 312-787-7200 (Walk 21)

Blackstone www.marriott.com, 636 S. Michigan Ave., 312-447-0955 (Walk 23)

Chicago Hilton and Towers www.chicagohilton.com, 720 S. Michigan Ave., 312-922-4400 (Walk 23)

Drake Hotel www.thedrakehotel.com, 140 E. Walton Pl., 312-787-2200 (Walk 20)

Hard Rock Hotel Carbon and Carbide Building www.hardrockhotelchicago.com, 30 N. Michigan Ave., 312-345-1000 (Walk 23)

Intercontinental Hotel www.icchicagohotel.com, 505 N. Michigan Ave., 312-944-4100 (Walk 20)

Reliance Building (a.k.a. Hotel Burnham, www.burnhamhotel.com, 312-782-1111) 1 W. Washington St. (Walk 17)

Natural areas and Parks

Belmont Harbor (Walk 26)

Burnham Park (Walk 5)

Erie Park (Walk 18)

Grant Park (Walk 6 and Walk 23)

Harrison Park (Walk 14)

Holstein Park 2200 N. Oakley Ave. (Walk 30)

Humboldt Park (Walk 29)

Jackson Park (Walk 2)

Lincoln Park (Walk 22 and Walk 25)

Millennium Park (Walk 16)

Montrose Harbor (Walk 26)

North Branch of the Chicago River 4200 N. to 4400 N. (Walk 26)

North Park Village Nature Center 5801 N. Pulaski Rd., 312-744-5472 (Walk 28)

Northerly Island (Walk 6)

Oz Park N. Lincoln Ave. and W. Webster Ave. (Walk 22)

Ping Tom Park (Walk 15)

Promontory Point (Walk 4)

Rainbow Beach Park 3111 E. 77th St., 312-745-1479 (Walk 1)

Washington Park (Walk 2)

Washington Square Park (Walk 18)

Welles Park N. Lincoln Ave. and W. Montrose Ave. (Walk 26)

Wicker Park 1425 N. Damen Ave. (Walk 31)

SHOPPING

57th Street Books 1301 E. 57th St., 773-684-1300 (Walk 3)

Abraham Lincoln Book Shop 357 W. Chicago Ave., 312-944-3085 (Walk 18)

Acala's 1733 W. Chicago Ave., 312-226-0152 (Walk 31)

Alchemy Arts 1203 W. Bryn Mawr Ave., 773-769-4970 (Walk 25)

All She Wrote 825 W. Armitage Ave., 773-529-0100 (Walk 22)

American Girl Place 111 E. Chicago Ave., 312-943-9400 (Walk 20)

Argo Georgian Bakery 2812 W. Devon Ave., 773-764-6322 (Walk 28)

Artesanias D' Mexico 1644 W. 18th St., 312-563-9779 (Walk 14)

Athenian Candle Company 300 S. Halsted St., 312-332-6988 (Walk 11)

Athens Grocery 324 S. Halsted St., 312-454-0940 (Walk 11)

Batteries Not Included 3420 N. Halsted St., 773-935-9900 (Walk 24)

BomBon Bakery 1508 W. 18th St., 312-733-7788 (Walk 14)

Book Cellar 4736 N. Lincoln Ave., 773-293-2665 (Walk 27)

Borders Bookstore 4718 N. Broadway, 773-334-7338 (Walk 25)

Brown Elephant 3651 N. Halsted St., 773-549-5943 (Walk 24)

Chirugi Hardware 1449 W. Taylor St., 312-666-2235 (Walk 12)

Conte Di Savoia 1438 W. Taylor St., 312-666-3471 (Walk 12)

Del Rey Tortilleria 1023 W. 18th St., 312-829-3725 (Walk 14)

Dig It! 11208 S. St. Lawrence Ave., 773-520-1373 (Walk 7)

Doolin's 511 N. Halsted St., 312-243-9424 (Walk 11)

Erickson's Deli 5250 N. Clark St., 773-561-5634 (Walk 25)

Flourish Bakery Cafe 1138 W. Bryn Mawr Ave., 773-271-2253 (Walk 25)

Fresh Farms International Market 2626 W. Devon Ave., 773-764-5757 (Walk 28)

G Boutique 2131 N. Damen Ave., 773-235-1234 (Walk 30)

Heads and Threads Boutique 1254 N. Milwaukee Ave., 773-235-1190 (Walk 31)

Hong Kong Noodle Co. 2350 S. Wentworth Ave., 312-842-0480 (Walk 15)

Hynes' Irish Cottage 1907 West 103rd St., 773-429-0666 (Walk 8)

India Book House 2551 W. Devon Ave., 866-656-5999 (Walk 28)

Intermix 841 W. Armitage Ave., 773-404-8766 (Walk 22)

Iqra Book Center 2749 W. Devon Ave., 773-274-2665 (Walk 28)

Jackson Park (Walk 2)

Jazz Record Mart 27 E. Illinois St., 312-222-1467 (Walk 18)

Kate the Greats 5550 N. Broadway, 773-561-1932 (Walk 25)

Lori's Shoes 824 W. Armitage Ave., 773-281-5655 (Walk 22)

Magic Tree Bookstore 141 N. Oak Park Ave., 708-848-0770 (Walk 9)

Marilyn Miglin Institute 112 E. Oak St., 800-662-1120 (Walk 21)

Merz Apothecary 4716 N. Lincoln Ave., 773-989-0900 (Walk 27)

Music House 2925 W. Devon Ave., 773-262-7309 (Walk 28)

Myopic Books 1468 N. Milwaukee Ave., 773-862-4882 (Walk 31)

N. Fagin Books 459 N. Milwaukee Ave., 312-829-5252 (Walk 11)

Nea Agora 1056 W. Taylor St., 312-271-2080 (Walk 12)

O'Gara & Wilson 1448 E. 57th St., 773-363-0993 (Walk 3)

Powell's Used Bookstore 1501 E. 57th St., 773-955-7780 (Walk 3)

Presence 5216 N. Clark St., 773-989-4420 (Walk 25)

Reckless Records 1532 N. Milwaukee Ave., 773-235-3727 (Walk 31)

Sandmeyer's Bookstore 714 S. Dearborn St., 312-922-2104 (Walk 17)

Scafuri Bakery 1337 W. Taylor St., 312-733-8881 (Walk 12)

Seminary Co-op Bookstore 5757 S. University Ave., 773-752-4381 (Walk 3)

Stadium Seat Store 4251 N. Lincoln Ave., 773-404-7975 (Walk 27)

Stitch 1723 N. Damen Ave., 773-782-1570 (Walk 30)

Sun Sun Tong 2260 S. Wentworth Ave., 312-842-6398 (Walk 15)

Ten Ren Tea and Ginseng 2247 S. Wentworth Ave., 312-842-1171 (Walk 15)

Thai Grocery 5014 N. Broadway, 773-561-5345 (Walk 25)

Three Sisters 2854 W. Devon Ave., 773-465-6695 (Walk 28)

Unabridged Books 3251 N. Broadway, 773-883-9119 (Walk 26)

University Market 1323 E. 57th St., 773-363-0070 (Walk 3)

Wolfbait and B-Girls 3131 W. Logan Blvd., 312-698-8685 (Walk 30)

Women and Children First 5233 N. Clark St., 773-769-9299 (Walk 25)

World Music Company www.worldfolkmusiccompany.com, 1808 W. 103rd St, 773-779-2546 (Walk 8)

Yin Wall 2112A S. Archer Ave., 312-225-2888 (Walk 15)

BOOKS & WEBSITES

AIA Guide to Chicago, 2nd ed., edited by Alice Sinkevitch (Harvest Books, 2004). The absolute bible for a city that worships architecture, with often tart commentary on some of the bigger duds on the skyline.

A Guide to Chicago's Murals, by Mary Lackritz Gray (University of Chicago Press, 2001). From hidden viaducts to private clubs, Gray finds the strange, moving, and joyous.

Hollywood on Lake Michigan, by Arnie Bernstein (Lake Claremont Press, 1998). As the subtitle says: "100 years of Chicago and the movies."

Never a City So Real, by Alex Kotlowitz (Crown, 2004). A savvy walk through the city by one of its best chroniclers.

Return to the Scene of the Crime, by Richard Lindberg (Cumberland House, 1999). Longtime local author literally digs up some of the more colorful examples of local mayhem.

Sidewalks: Portraits of Chicago, by Rick Kogan and Charles Osgood (Northwestern University Press, 2006). A compendium of the popular *Chicago Tribune* feature brings to life the kinds of people you'll meet while using this book.

Sin in the Second City, by Karen Abbott (Random House, 2007). A stimulating look at Chicago's lurid legacy.

Streetwise Chicago, by Don Hayner and Tom McNamee (Wild Onion Books, 1988). A comprehensive guide to the history of Chicago street names. Where else would you learn that Carpenter Street isn't named for the trade but rather Philo Carpenter, a 19th-century local humanitarian?

Beachwood Reporter, www.beachwoodreporter.com. Insightful and often biting commentary on Chicago politics and media.

Encyclopedia of Chicago, encyclopedia.chicagohistory.org. A great resource, with articles by local scholars and luminaries. Look for the interactive features like the plan of the city.

Forgotten Chicago, www.forgottenchicago.com. Long-lost aspects of the city are recalled at this smart site.

Gaper's Block, www.gapersblock.com. Named for the clichéd stalwart of Chicago traffic news, this site combines news, commentary and fun from a wide range of contributors.

INDEX

(*Italicized* page numbers
indicate photos.)

about the author

Ryan Ver Berkmoes never tires of walking Chicago. Who could? Starting in 1983 when he walked home for the first time to his minute studio in Lincoln Park from his shabby Loop office, he has never tired of the infinite surprises encountered on the city's streets. One time it was running into a bunch of Vietnam vets in Grant Park at 2 AM who were with the traveling Vietnam War Memorial and over shared pizza broke his heart with their tales of sacrifice. Another time it was wandering out to the end of the North Ave. Beach breakwater at dawn and being struck by the incomparable beauty of the often-seen skyline. Still another time it was bumping into an old friend on a North Side street and catching up— and falling down—during an impromptu pub crawl.

During his years living in Chicago, Ryan wrote in one way or another for pretty much every publication with the name Chicago in it. He's also lived around the world and written books from places as diverse as Bali, Sri Lanka, Russia and Ireland. But he always returns to Chicago and is sorry he ever saw an old tourism ad hyping the city in 1983, which featured Mike Ditka and Dick Butkus meeting at Butch McGuire's while the sappy, syrupy song "Calling me home Chicago" swelled in the background. Even now, whether arriving by plane, train or car, and feeling a pang of emotion as he returns to the place he considers home, that damn song starts playing in his head.

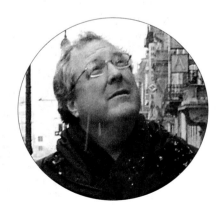